HOW
SEX
WORKS

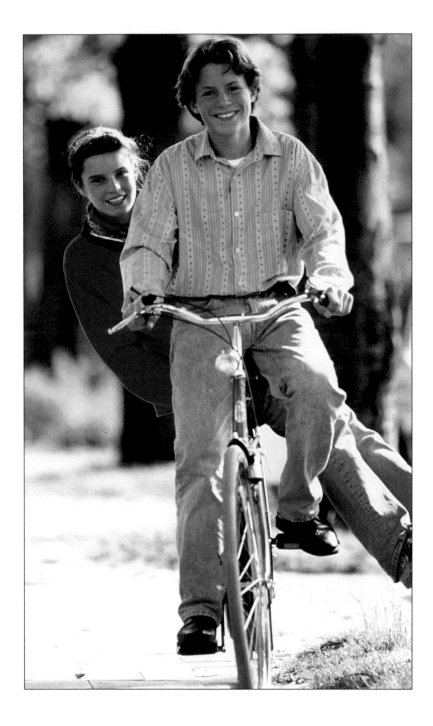

HOW SEX WORKS

A clear, comprehensive guide for teenagers to emotional, physical, and sexual maturity

Elizabeth Fenwick
& Richard Walker

A DK PUBLISHING BOOK

Project editor Charyn Jones
U.S. editor Mary Ann Lynch
Art editor Ursula Dawson
Deputy editorial director Daphne Razazan
Managing art editor Derek Coombes

First American Edition, 1994
4 6 8 10 9 7 5 3
Published in the United States by DK Publishing, Inc.,
95 Madison Avenue, New York, New York 10016

Library of Congress Cataloging-in-Publication Data

Fenwick, Elizabeth.
How sex works: a clear, comprehensive guide for teenagers to emotional, physical, and
sexual maturity / by Elizabeth Fenwick and Richard Walker. -- 1st American ed.
p.   cm.
Includes index.
ISBN 1-56458-505-0
ISBN 0-7894-0634-9 (paper)
1. Sex. 2. Sex instruction for teenagers -- United States.
3. Teenagers -- United States -- Sexual behavior. 4. Hygiene, Sexual.
I. Walker, Richard.
II. Title.
HQ35.F39   1994
613.9'0835--dc20   93-37638   CIP
Reproduced by J. Film Process Pte., Thailand
Printed in Hong Kong by Wing King Tong Co. Ltd.

CONTENTS

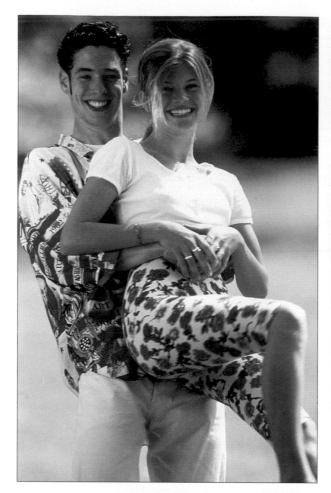

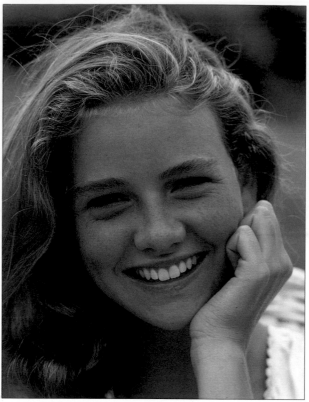

BECOMING AN ADULT
Preparing yourself for relationships is crucial.
Relationships don't just happen; making and sustaining
them is a skill that everyone needs to learn.

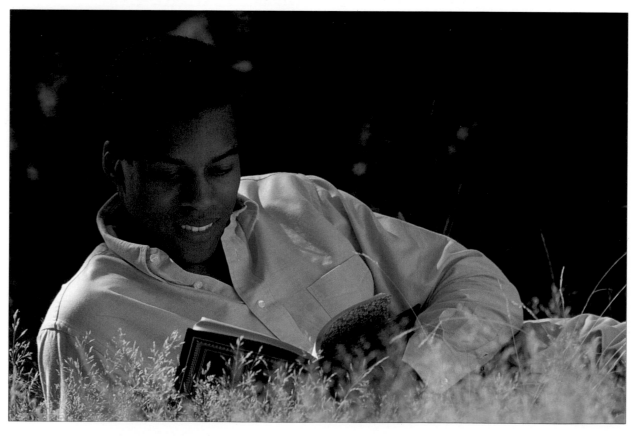

INTRODUCTION

There is probably no more sensitive or controversial topic involving teenagers today than their sexual lives. In the discussion of whether teenagers "should" or "should not" be sexually active, other important aspects of growing up are often overlooked. Becoming sexually active is just one aspect of becoming an adult. *How Sex Works* is a guide for teens to all aspects of growing up – emotional, physical, and sexual. Our aim throughout has been to provide straight answers to all the kinds of questions a young person naturally has. Every section is clearly illustrated, so that the reader can see, as well as read about, the body in different stages.

Each person develops at such different rates that "Am I normal?" is probably one of the most common questions teens want to ask. The introductory section, "Understanding the Body," addresses this question, covering the major physical changes a teen can expect, and including illustrations of both the male and female reproductive systems. "Relationships and Emotions" focuses on feelings, social life, and friends, acknowledging that various cultural and religious backgrounds also influence young people's developing values. "What Happens During Sex" explains what sex is actually like, providing clear, illustrated answers to the sorts of questions the average teen has. "Contraception" covers the various methods of contraception available and how to use them properly. How pregnancy starts, childbirth, and unplanned pregnancy are included in the section "Pregnancy and Being a Parent." "Sex and Health" features a comprehensive list of sexually transmitted diseases as well as a section on HIV/AIDS, and general information on taking care of one's body. Sex and the law, sexual harassment, child abuse, and rape are included in "Problem Areas," followed by a list of useful addresses.

We hope that every reader, male and female, will read the entire book. The best decisions are those based upon the most complete information possible. And where sexual health is concerned, it is just as important to know and understand one's partner as it is to know and understand oneself. Knowing about sex doesn't mean you have to have sex; rather, it should give you the confidence to proceed at your own rate, and not be rushed into having a sexual relationship just because someone else wants you to.

Whether the decision is to postpone sexual activity until marriage or the post-teen years, or to become sexually active at an earlier time, every teen needs to take responsibility for his or her own sexual activity and sexual health. Every sexual action carries with it consequences. No one can afford to assume that the other person will be the one to make sure sex is handled in the "safest" possible way. In covering the many aspects of growing to adulthood, *How Sex Works* provides information for teenagers trying not only to understand themselves and their friends, but to chart their way through problems never dreamed of in earlier generations.

UNDERSTANDING THE BODY

Becoming a woman

Between the ages of 10 and 18, the female body changes from that of a child to that of a woman. The shape becomes more rounded, the waist narrows, the breasts and hips develop, and the weight almost doubles.

The way a person looks is determined mainly by what they inherit from their parents. When the mother's egg and the father's sperm met during fertilization (*see page 70*), each was carrying a package of information consisting of thousands of genes. These packages fused to provide a complete set of pairs of genes. Each pair controls, or helps control, one of the body's features, such as skin color, breast size, and height. A gene inherited from the mother may be stronger than one from the father, or the other way around. For example, if a baby inherited a brown-eyed gene from the mother, and a blue-eyed gene from the father, that baby will probably have brown eyes because brown is a dominant color.

Bodies don't differ just because of inherited characteristics, however. Lifestyle can make a difference as well. Some people eat a lot, and their metabolism makes them put on weight; whereas others might eat the same amount and not gain weight. A well-balanced diet and exercise contribute to maintaining a weight appropriate to one's body type.

PERSONAL HYGIENE

At around 12 or 13, sweat glands in the armpits start to work. Everyone sweats when they exercise or are excited or nervous – some more than others. Fresh sweat doesn't smell; its characteristic odor develops after a few hours. A daily bath or shower is important, and so is a deodorant that covers the smell. For those who sweat heavily, there are deodorants combined with an antiperspirant to reduce sweating. Shaving the armpits and legs is a matter of personal choice. Shaving and hair-removal creams can inflame the skin for a few hours so it is best not to apply a deodorant immediately after removing hair. Shaving is an easy way to remove unwanted hair, though hair removal creams (depilatories) and waxing are also effective methods.

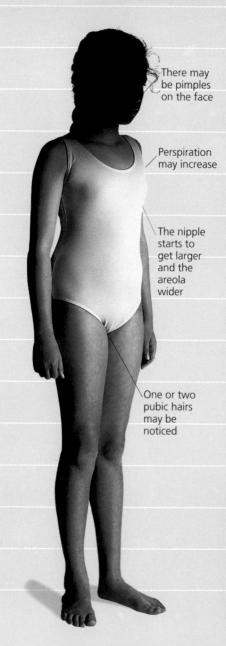

GROWING UP
Until the age of 10 or 11, children grow steadily and slowly. But as puberty begins, growth accelerates. This growth spurt usually starts two years earlier in girls than it does in boys (*see page 20*) and lasts about a year. Growth continues at a steady rate until, by the age of 18, adult height and shape have been reached.

There may be pimples on the face

Perspiration may increase

The nipple starts to get larger and the areola wider

One or two pubic hairs may be noticed

12 years
Height: 4 ft 6 in/137 cm
Weight: 70 lb/32 kg

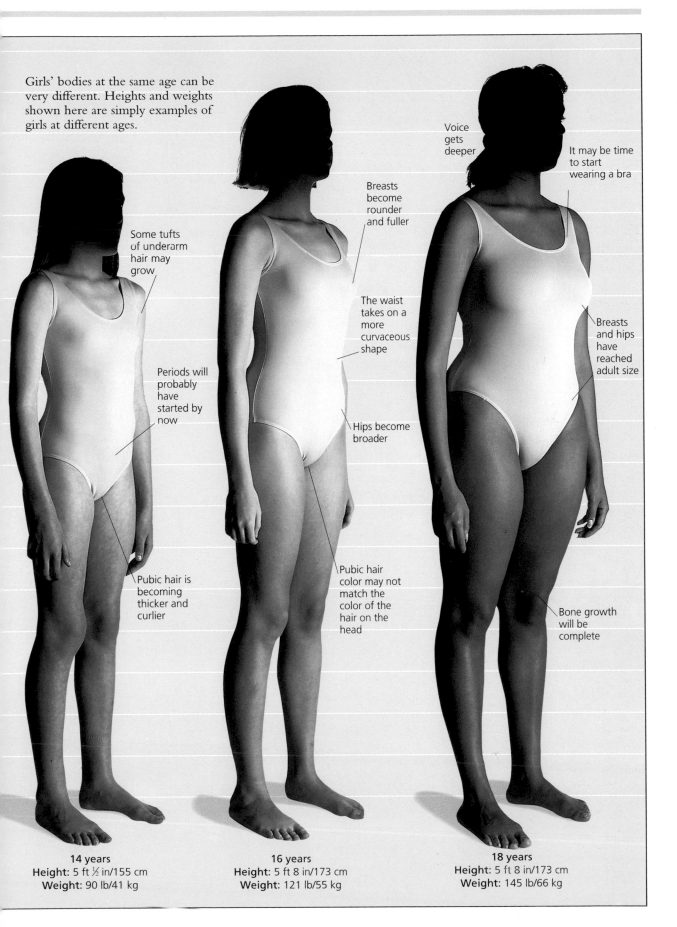

Girls' bodies at the same age can be very different. Heights and weights shown here are simply examples of girls at different ages.

Some tufts of underarm hair may grow

Periods will probably have started by now

Pubic hair is becoming thicker and curlier

Breasts become rounder and fuller

The waist takes on a more curvaceous shape

Hips become broader

Pubic hair color may not match the color of the hair on the head

Voice gets deeper

It may be time to start wearing a bra

Breasts and hips have reached adult size

Bone growth will be complete

14 years
Height: 5 ft ½ in/155 cm
Weight: 90 lb/41 kg

16 years
Height: 5 ft 8 in/173 cm
Weight: 121 lb/55 kg

18 years
Height: 5 ft 8 in/173 cm
Weight: 145 lb/66 kg

A girl at puberty

Puberty is the time during which the female body starts to change from a child's body to that of a woman. The changes do not begin at the same age for every girl, and the speed of change varies, too.

The changes that occur during puberty happen because of the increase in the levels of the female sex hormones estrogen and progesterone (*see page 16*). Puberty generally starts earlier in girls than in boys, usually around the age of 10 or 11, although it may begin before or after this age. Each person, male or female, has his or her biological time clock. As the body changes, so, too, will feelings and attitudes.

Some will notice that they are growing more rapidly – this is known as a growth spurt. Some girls find themselves taller than many of the boys in their class. Breasts start developing now; strands of hair may grow on the pubic area (*see page 14*) and under the armpits; hips, thighs, and breasts become more rounded. Periods may begin, too (*see page 17*).

The skin secretes more oil

Perspiration glands become more active

The areola – the darker skin around the nipple – gets wider and darker

The hips start to become fleshier

Thighs develop

A few pubic hairs may grow on the mons pubis or around the labia

The internal organs also have a growth spurt during puberty

A GIRL AT PUBERTY

EATING WELL

The attitude that thin is beautiful is widespread in some cultures; in the western world, it has been found that almost every woman diets at some time in her life. There may be a real sense of achievement when weight is lost. However, it is obvious that not everyone grows up to look like a model in a magazine – thin and tall. For some girls, being thin becomes an obsession. Anorexia is an illness in which the sufferer sees herself as fat and continues to diet and perhaps exercise in an attempt to lose more weight. Even though she may be painfully thin, this will not be her perception of herself. Her weight may drop dramatically, and her periods may stop. Some anorexics starve themselves to death. Some develop bulimia, which is maintaining a normal weight by "binge eating" and then making themselves vomit the food up. People with these eating disorders need help, not just to get back to a healthier eating pattern, but because the disorder is usually a sign of underlying unhappiness. Those with anorexia or bulimia need medical attention but may also benefit from counseling.

DIFFERENCES IN GROWTH

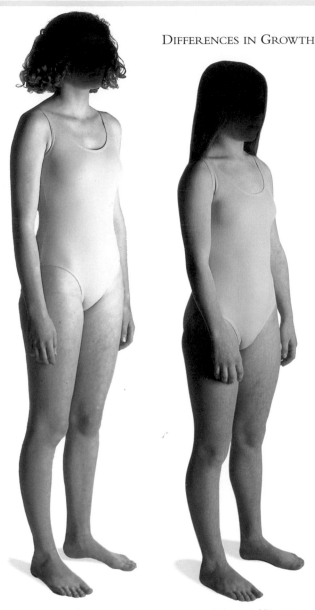
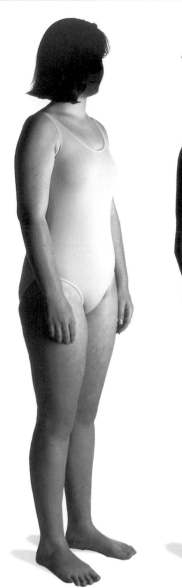
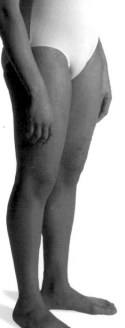

Height: 5 ft 9 in/175 cm
Weight: 125 lb/57 kg

Height: 5 ft ½ in/155 cm
Weight: 97 lb/44 kg

Height: 5 ft 8 in/173 cm
Weight: 147 lb/67 kg

Height: 5 ft 3 in/162 cm
Weight: 112 lb/51 kg

RATES OF GROWTH

Although changes to the body shape and size happen in a fairly orderly way, all girls develop at different rates. Some girls may experience a growth spurt at 11; others may not notice any difference in height until they are 13. It is also at the time of this growth spurt that the body changes become noticeable and the first period occurs. The girls pictured here are 13 and all aged within six months of one another.

QUESTIONS AND ANSWERS

I seem to get pimples just when I really want to look good. Would it help if I stopped eating chocolate?
Schula, 14 years

There is no conclusive evidence that diet impacts acne, although some may find certain foods aggravate skin eruptions. It is high levels of sex hormones that lead to acne during adolescence. Washing your face regularly may help. If the acne is bad, see a dermatologist, who may prescribe an oral medication or a gel.

My breasts are small, but my friend says I still ought to wear a bra, or the muscles will get weak. Do I have to?
Sally, 13 years

Breasts have no muscles. Large breasts may droop without a bra. The time to start wearing a bra is probably when you start to feel uncomfortable without one. Special sports bras are available for those needing extra support when involved in exercise or sports.

The female body

The reproductive system in the female body, including the eggs in the ovaries, is in place at birth. A signal in the brain at the onset of puberty starts the fertile stage of your life, causing one egg to be released every month until around the age of about 50.

Each month, one egg matures and is released into one of the fallopian tubes. If sperm are there after recent sexual intercourse (*see pages 70-71*), the egg may be fertilized. The tubes lead to the uterus where the baby grows. The neck of the uterus is called the cervix. This has a mucous plug that thins at ovulation (when an egg is released), making it easier for sperm to swim through. The vagina is an elastic tube running to the opening at the vulva. It is quite separate from the urinary system, which has its own opening – the urethra.

The uterus is about the size and shape of a pear. It is the most muscular organ in the body and it is capable of huge expansion. It usually tilts forward, almost at a right angle to the vagina. Its lower part, the cervix, opens into the vagina, and the tip of the cervix can just be felt at the top of the vagina.

During puberty (*see page 12*), the external sexual organs develop and mature. The mons pubis – the pad of fat covering the pubic bone – becomes fleshier and more prominent. Pubic hair grows on the labia.

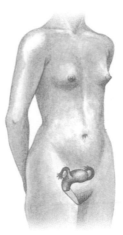

THE PELVIS
The reproductive organs lie in the pelvis (body cage) where they are protected. The uterus lies above and behind the bladder and in front of the rectum.

THE VULVA
Between two outer fleshy lips, or labia, on which the pubic hair grows, are two thinner and hairless inner labia. Between these are the clitoris, at the front; the opening of the urethra, in the middle; and the larger vaginal opening behind that.

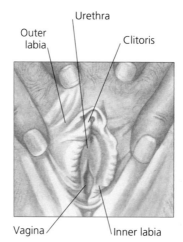

Outer labia

Urethra

Clitoris

Vagina

Inner labia

THE STRUCTURE OF THE BREASTS

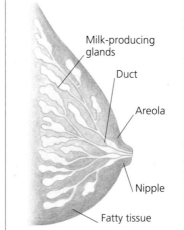

Milk-producing glands

Duct

Areola

Nipple

Fatty tissue

Breasts are made up of fatty tissue containing tiny milk-producing glands. All women have a similar number of glands, but some have more fatty tissue than others. This is why some breasts are larger than others. Ducts run from the glands to the surface of the nipple. The nipple is the most sensitive part of the breast. It is soft, but cold, and both touch and sexual arousal make it hard and erect. Around the nipple is the areola, an area of pink or brown skin, which darkens with age and during pregnancy. During pregnancy the milk-producing ducts increase in preparation for lactation. They replace much of the fat that is normally in the breast. Milk is produced inside the glands when a woman has had a baby. The milk travels through the ducts to the nipple as the baby sucks.

Fimbriae lie near the surface of the ovary and receive eggs

At birth, the ovaries contain about 400,000 eggs, or ova, in sacs called follicles. One egg is released each month. The empty follicle develops into the corpus luteum. Ovaries also produce the female sex hormones, estrogen and progesterone

The inside of a fallopian tube is no wider than the diameter of a human hair. Cells in the tubes sweep eggs to the uterus. If sperm are present, fertilization may take place in the tube

Bladder

Clitoris

Urethra

The vagina is about 3 in (8 cm) long, with ridged walls. These normally lie against each other, but because they are elastic, they can open during intercourse and stretch in childbirth. In childhood, the vaginal opening is partially covered by a membrane called the hymen

FROM OVARY TO UTERUS

At its upper end, the uterus opens out into the fallopian tubes, whose fringed ends lie near the surface of the ovaries. In this illustration, the fallopian tubes and ovaries are shown larger than life size; in reality, an ovary is about 1¼ in (3 cm) long, and the eggs in it are minute. The fallopian tube is about ⅟₂₅ in (1 mm) thick.

The uterus is a hollow, pear-shaped, muscular organ. It is capable of huge expansion to accommodate a baby

The cervix, the neck of the uterus, leads to the vagina. It is plugged with mucus, with only a small hole to allow blood to pass through during periods. However, at ovulation, the mucus thins, making it easier for sperm to enter the uterus

Rectum

QUESTIONS AND ANSWERS

If you're a virgin, is your vagina completely closed?
Rebecca, 14 years

No. A membrane called a hymen surrounds the vaginal opening, but only very rarely does it block the whole opening. There is normally a hole in it at least big enough to allow the menstrual blood to flow out. The hymen is eventually torn or stretched by vigorous exercise, using tampons, or sexual intercourse.

What happens to the eggs that don't get used?
Jan, 13 years

Out of the 400,000 eggs present in your ovaries at birth, probably only about 400 mature to be released at ovulation. The rest fail to mature and are reabsorbed into your body. When there are no more eggs to be released, menopause occurs.

Someone told me twins happen because of something in the

woman's system, and that they run in families. Is this true?
Adam, 14 years

Fraternal twins do tend to run in families. If a woman's ovaries shed two eggs at once and if they are both fertilized, she will have fraternal twins. These twins are not identical and may be different sexes. Identical twins develop when one egg is fertilized by a single sperm and the egg divides to form two babies. These twins are the same sex and look alike.

The menstrual cycle

If an egg is not fertilized by sperm on its voyage down the fallopian tube, the lining of the uterus, which has prepared itself for the egg, is shed through the vagina. This monthly shedding of the lining of the uterus is called menstruation, or a period.

Periods are the sign that hormones have stimulated the ovaries to begin releasing eggs. They also mean that the body is physically able to have a baby. First periods usually begin between the ages of 11 and 14, but some girls start as early as nine and others not until they are 16.

The blood that comes out through the vagina is often scant at first, and for the first six months it may not be bright red, but brownish. There may be just a trickle the first day, a heavier flow during the second and third day, then less and less until the discharge is back to normal on the fifth or sixth day. For the first two days, there may be some discomfort, with abdominal cramps. This is quite common.

The menstrual cycle may be irregular for a while – periods may be missed – but after a few months, there will be a regular pattern. The average length of the menstrual cycle (from the first day of one period to the first day of the next) is 28 days, but all women have slightly different cycles.

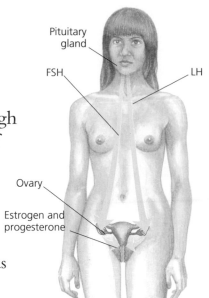

Pituitary gland

FSH

LH

Ovary

Estrogen and progesterone

HORMONAL CONTROL
The events of the menstrual cycle are controlled by hormones. Follicle-stimulating hormone (FSH) and luteinizing hormone (LH), released by the pituitary gland in the brain, are carried by the bloodstream to the ovary. Here they cause an egg to ripen and be released, and the ovary to release another two hormones, estrogen and progesterone, that thicken the lining of the uterus, or endometrium.

DYSMENORRHEA

This is the medical word for very painful periods. The lower abdominal pains are called cramps, and they feel as if something is pulling the body inside. Painkillers can help. Some girls become bloated, some depressed, some feel very ill, and some even vomit. If period symptoms are particularly severe, a doctor may prescribe a drug that will relieve the symptoms. Dysmenorrhea can be treated successfully. The pains usually get less as one gets older, or they may decrease if one is using contraceptive pills. Exercise or yoga can also help relieve the discomfort.

QUESTIONS AND ANSWERS

Is it true you can't get pregnant before your periods have started?
Simone, 13 years

No. In theory you could, because your period might be about to start. However, usually no egg is released during the first few menstrual cycles.

How do I know when I'm likely to start having my period?
Alison, 14 years

Your period won't start until your growth spurt has begun and your breasts and pubic hair are growing. Starting early or late runs in families: if your mother started her periods late, you may, too. You may notice some whitish discharge for about a year before the bleeding begins.

Some girls at school stay out of gym when they have their period. Will I need to do this?
Connie, 14 years

You can do anything during your period that you do at any other time. Depression, irritability, pimples, headaches, swollen or tender breasts, and stomach cramps are symptoms that some women get during their period. When these symptoms occur before your period, they are known as premenstrual syndrome (PMS). Whatever the symptom, you need to find a remedy that works for you. One of the best remedies for cramps, for example, is a hot water bottle. There are also painkillers, especially for menstrual or premenstrual pain.

THE MENSTRUAL CYCLE

Although the average length of the menstrual cycle is 28 days, the variation in the length of a cycle can be anything from 21 to 42 days. However long the menstrual cycle is in days, ovulation occurs 12 to 16 days *before* the beginning of the next period. If the egg is not fertilized, the uterine lining is shed through the vagina. During the cycle, the cervical mucus also changes. This can be used as an indication of ovulation (*see page 68*).

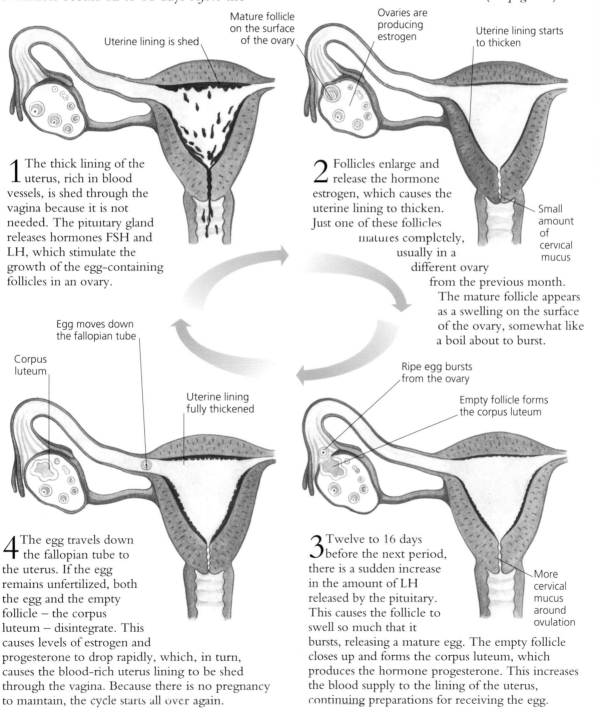

1 The thick lining of the uterus, rich in blood vessels, is shed through the vagina because it is not needed. The pituitary gland releases hormones FSH and LH, which stimulate the growth of the egg-containing follicles in an ovary.

Uterine lining is shed

Mature follicle on the surface of the ovary

2 Follicles enlarge and release the hormone estrogen, which causes the uterine lining to thicken. Just one of these follicles matures completely, usually in a different ovary from the previous month. The mature follicle appears as a swelling on the surface of the ovary, somewhat like a boil about to burst.

Ovaries are producing estrogen

Uterine lining starts to thicken

Small amount of cervical mucus

4 The egg travels down the fallopian tube to the uterus. If the egg remains unfertilized, both the egg and the empty follicle – the corpus luteum – disintegrate. This causes levels of estrogen and progesterone to drop rapidly, which, in turn, causes the blood-rich uterus lining to be shed through the vagina. Because there is no pregnancy to maintain, the cycle starts all over again.

Corpus luteum

Egg moves down the fallopian tube

Uterine lining fully thickened

3 Twelve to 16 days before the next period, there is a sudden increase in the amount of LH released by the pituitary. This causes the follicle to swell so much that it bursts, releasing a mature egg. The empty follicle closes up and forms the corpus luteum, which produces the hormone progesterone. This increases the blood supply to the lining of the uterus, continuing preparations for receiving the egg.

Ripe egg bursts from the ovary

Empty follicle forms the corpus luteum

More cervical mucus around ovulation

Monthly periods

No one knows quite why menstruation starts, but we do know that around 9 to 16 years a gland in the brain triggers the process by releasing hormones. These in turn stimulate the ovaries to produce the female sex hormones that encourage the body to change.

For past generations of women, menstruation was an unmentionable, and in some cultures a time when women were seen as unclean. Today, with more open attitudes toward sexuality, girls can feel proud realizing that menstruation signals their entry into womanhood. Even so, many girls still start their periods without ever having been told what to expect.

Having a period is a completely normal part of a woman's life, but it is understandable for girls to feel embarrassed and uncomfortable when they first begin. This may depend upon how helpful and supportive their parents are. Girls often worry that they may smell, or that blood will leak onto their clothes and everyone will know what is happening to them. Girlfriends will understand these feelings, but boys may be insensitive and make jokes. Knowing what to expect helps ease initial embarrassment.

Some find it a good idea to keep track of their periods so that they can see how their personal cycle develops. It is then possible to know what to expect.

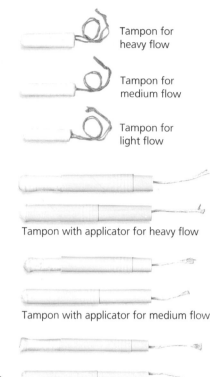

Tampon for heavy flow

Tampon for medium flow

Tampon for light flow

Tampon with applicator for heavy flow

Tampon with applicator for medium flow

Tampon with applicator for light flow

TAMPONS

A tampon is a tight roll of cotton fiber with a string at one end. Tampons are available in different thicknesses to suit the rate of flow. If there are leaks, then use either a higher absorbency tampon, change the tampon more often, or use a napkin during the heavier flow of your period. A tampon cannot get lost inside or be put in the wrong opening.

PERSONAL HYGIENE

Good personal hygiene is particularly important during a period. The area around the vagina should be washed, but not inside – the lining is sensitive. A daily bath or shower is the best approach to keeping clean and warding off odors. Scented bubble baths and oils may also cause irritation. It is important to change tampons frequently – at least four times a day – to prevent the growth of bacteria in the vagina. This can lead to a condition called toxic shock syndrome (*see page 64*).

SANITARY NAPKINS

Sanitary napkins are soft cotton pads with one waterproof side. They are used to absorb menstrual blood and are worn outside the body, unlike tampons. Napkins come in thicknesses suited to the rate of flow, which varies over the course of a period. They adhere to the lining of panties; some have wing shapes to hold them more firmly and provide for a heavier flow and prevent staining. Napkins should be changed several times a day. Some women prefer napkins when there is spotting rather than a steady flow and at night.

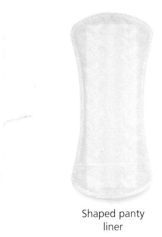

Panty liner with wings

Shaped panty liner

INSERTING A TAMPON

Tampons are worn inside the vagina, inserted with an applicator or with a finger. They are convenient for sports and can be worn during swimming. Low-absorbency tampons are useful when there is spotting rather than a steady flow.

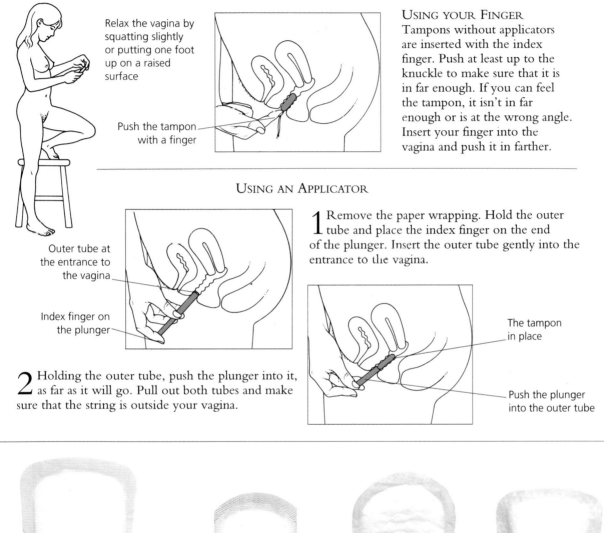

Relax the vagina by squatting slightly or putting one foot up on a raised surface

Push the tampon with a finger

USING YOUR FINGER

Tampons without applicators are inserted with the index finger. Push at least up to the knuckle to make sure that it is in far enough. If you can feel the tampon, it isn't in far enough or is at the wrong angle. Insert your finger into the vagina and push it in farther.

USING AN APPLICATOR

Outer tube at the entrance to the vagina

Index finger on the plunger

1 Remove the paper wrapping. Hold the outer tube and place the index finger on the end of the plunger. Insert the outer tube gently into the entrance to the vagina.

2 Holding the outer tube, push the plunger into it, as far as it will go. Pull out both tubes and make sure that the string is outside your vagina.

The tampon in place

Push the plunger into the outer tube

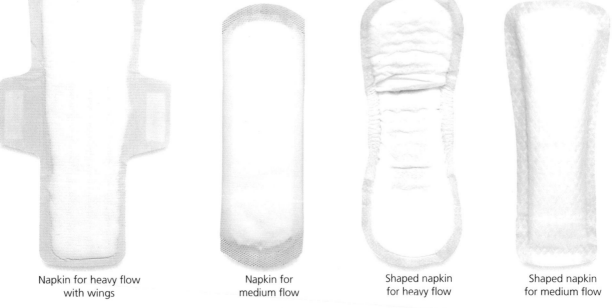

Napkin for heavy flow with wings

Napkin for medium flow

Shaped napkin for heavy flow

Shaped napkin for medium flow

Becoming a man

Between the ages of 13 and 18, the male body changes from that of a child to that of a man. The weight almost doubles, and the height increases. However, no two boys change in precisely the same way at the same age.

As a boy develops into a man, hair starts to grow and the voice becomes deeper. This changing voice can be embarrassing, because one minute it is a deep voice, and the next it is high and squeaky. What a person looks like depends a lot on what their parents look like and the genes they inherit from them (*see page 10*). Boys whose fathers have a lot of body hair will probably also have a lot. Body development also depends on factors such as exercise and diet.

Every boy is different, and physical changes in some boys may start at age 12, while other boys will develop even later. Many boys worry that they are developing too slowly or too quickly. It is easy to tease someone because they are bigger and hairier, or smaller and less hairy, than everyone else. However, everyone will eventually go through the same changes, although no two boys will look exactly alike.

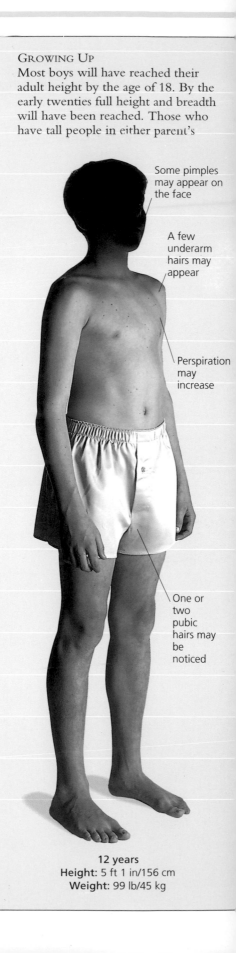

GROWING UP
Most boys will have reached their adult height by the age of 18. By the early twenties full height and breadth will have been reached. Those who have tall people in either parent's

Some pimples may appear on the face

A few underarm hairs may appear

Perspiration may increase

One or two pubic hairs may be noticed

12 years
Height: 5 ft 1 in/156 cm
Weight: 99 lb/45 kg

QUESTIONS AND ANSWERS

My friends have started laughing about me and saying that I smell. What can I do?
William, 14 years

Many things about your body change as you grow up. One of these is that you start to sweat more and your sweat has a different smell. A bath or shower every day is the best safeguard against odor. Wear clean clothes and socks whenever possible. Use deodorant or an antiperspirant; you can buy these in supermarkets and drugstores.

What should I do about the fluffy hair on my face?
Ben, 15 years

The first facial hair is easily and safely removed using soap and water, or shaving foam, and a disposable razor. This first facial hair is not thick enough yet to be removed with an electric shaver.

My breasts have started to swell, and they are quite sore under the nipples. Am I going to change into a girl?
Adam, 15 years

No. This happens in quite a few boys of your age and is nothing to worry about. It is caused by a reaction to the sex hormones that are causing all the changes in your body, and it should not last more than a few months.

family may also be tall. Heights and weights shown here are simply examples of boys at different ages.

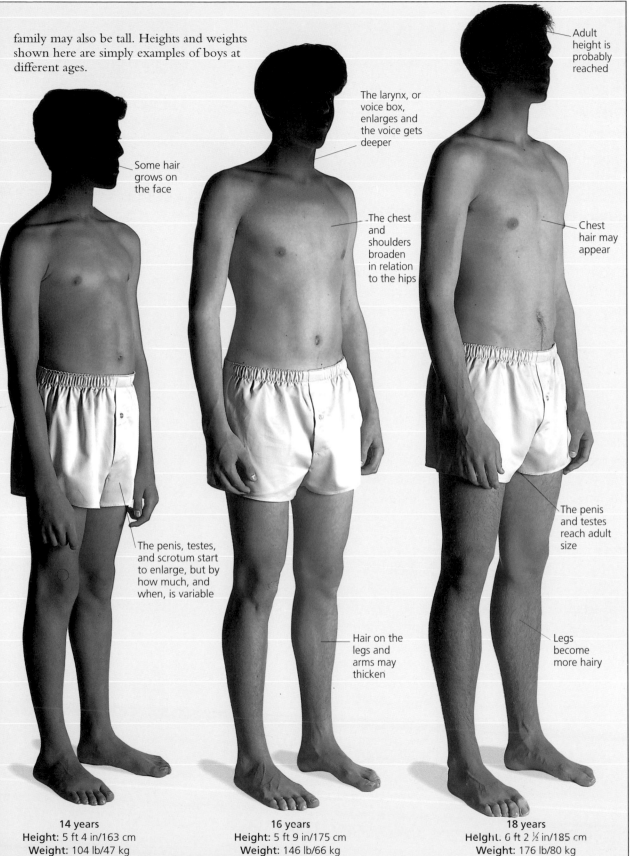

Some hair grows on the face

The larynx, or voice box, enlarges and the voice gets deeper

The chest and shoulders broaden in relation to the hips

Adult height is probably reached

Chest hair may appear

The penis, testes, and scrotum start to enlarge, but by how much, and when, is variable

The penis and testes reach adult size

Hair on the legs and arms may thicken

Legs become more hairy

14 years
Height: 5 ft 4 in/163 cm
Weight: 104 lb/47 kg

16 years
Height: 5 ft 9 in/175 cm
Weight: 146 lb/66 kg

18 years
Height: 6 ft 2 ½ in/185 cm
Weight: 176 lb/80 kg

A boy at puberty

Puberty is the time of life when a boy starts to become sexually mature. The reproductive organs develop, and the testes start producing sperm. The body begins a phase of growth and change in shape that will continue until the late teens.

Puberty is triggered by a hormone released by the pituitary gland in the brain. This stimulates the testes to release the male sex hormone, testosterone. This controls the changes happening to the body. Puberty starts later in boys than girls, usually around the age of 14, although it may begin before or after this age. Puberty does not happen overnight. It forms part of the transition from boy to man called adolescence. This is a time of overall growth: as the body matures, feelings and attitudes change as well (*see pages 30-31*).

THE MAJOR CHANGES

By the age of 13 or 14, some bodily changes will probably be noticeable. There may be differences in the age at which the different stages of change happen. First, the testes start to grow. As they do so, the scrotum (the bag containing the testes) expands, hangs low, and gets more wrinkly. The scrotum's skin gets redder in color in those who have fair skin, or darker in those who have dark skin; it also becomes thicker. A few pubic hairs grow around the place where the penis joins the body, and some hair may grow under the armpits.

The penis starts growing longer and thicker, and the skin color also darkens. The testes and scrotum continue enlarging, and one testis, usually the left, hangs lower. Tiny bumps appear on the skin of the scrotum and sometimes the penis, showing where hair may grow. Pubic hair will eventually spread upward and to the sides and become thicker and more curly. The body starts its growth spurt, getting larger and heavier, with broader shoulders and narrower hips.

The body sweats more, and it will be necessary to wash more often and use deodorants and antiperspirants to avoid body odors. Pimples might appear, usually on the chin or nose, which is the area on the face where the skin secretes the most oils.

The skin secretes more oil

Sweat glands become more active

Some hair growth under the arms

A few pubic hairs appear at the base of the penis

The body starts to grow taller

A BOY AT PUBERTY

DIFFERENCES IN GROWTH

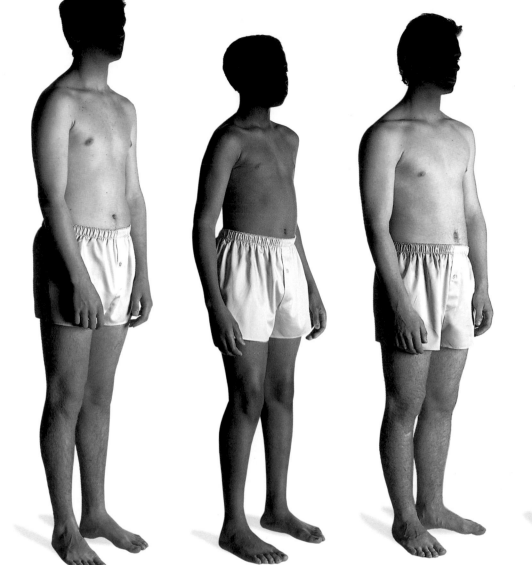

Height: 6 ft ½ in/183 cm
Weight: 154 lb/70 kg

Height: 5 ft 6 in/167 cm
Weight: 128 lb/58 kg

Height: 5 ft 10 in/178 cm
Weight: 167 lb/76 kg

Height: 5 ft 9 in/175 cm
Weight: 139 lb/63 kg

LOOKING AT DIFFERENCES

Everyone is different, both in the rate of the changes they experience, and in the shape and size they eventually reach at adulthood. This is partly inheritance from one's parents. Some may feel gawky and unattractive, or smaller and less hairy than their friends – everyone has some feature that they are embarrassed about. The boys pictured here are all 15 or 16 years old and aged within six months of one another.

QUESTIONS AND ANSWERS

I've started getting pimples. Why?
Jason, 14 years

Testosterone also makes the skin produce extra oils. Sometimes the glands in the skin that produce these oils get blocked, and pimples appear. Keep your skin clean with an antibacterial soap, and don't pick the pimples; you may get scarring. If they are really bad, you may have a condition called acne, and your doctor or dermatologist should be consulted.

How big should a penis be? My friends' all look much bigger than mine. It makes me really depressed.
Bobby, 15 years

Ask any male what part of his body he feels most unhappy about, and he will probably say the size of his penis, whatever age he is. A fully grown penis is usually between 3-4 in (8-10 cm) long when soft, and between 5-7 in (12-18 cm) long when it is erect, or stiff.

Male reproductive system

The male reproductive system isn't just a penis and testes that lie outside the body. Inside the body there is a system of ducts and glands that play an essential part in sperm production and delivery. Sperm are the male sex cells needed to make a baby.

From puberty to old age, millions of sperm are formed every day in the testes. It takes about 70 days for a sperm to be produced. Sperm can't develop properly at normal body temperature, so the testes hang outside the body, in the cooler scrotum. From the testis, sperm pass into a tube at the back of each testis – the epididymis – where the sperm mature. When a man ejaculates, muscle contractions squeeze the sperm along the sperm duct and into the urethra, passing on the way, the openings of the seminal vesicles and the prostate gland. These produce seminal fluids, which mobilize the sperm and make up the bulk of the semen that is ejaculated from the penis.

The shaft of the penis contains spongy erectile tissue, which fills with blood during an erection. The head, or glans, is highly sensitive. Sperm are ejaculated from the penis along the urethra. This is normally a channel for urine, but muscles at the bladder entrance contract during erection, so that no urine enters the semen, and no semen enters the bladder. Any sperm that are not ejaculated are reabsorbed within a certain time into the man's body.

MALE HORMONE

Testosterone is the male sex hormone that is made in the testes, and is needed for sperm production. During puberty, it also:
◼ Enlarges the penis, testes, and scrotum, and increases their sensitivity.
◼ Promotes growth and increases muscle bulk in the body.
◼ Stimulates growth of facial and bodily hair.
◼ Deepens the voice.
◼ Increases skin thickness and oily skin secretions, causing pimples.
◼ Increases a boy's sex drive and interest in sexual activity.

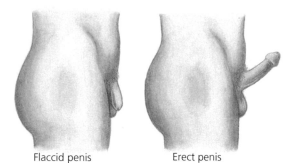

Flaccid penis   Erect penis

ERECTIONS AND SIZE DIFFERENCES
The penis hangs down, but during sexual arousal it becomes larger and points outward and upward, designed to deposit sperm in the vagina. Penises vary in size; size has nothing to do with masculinity, sexual performance, or pleasure.

CIRCUMCISION

Boys are born with a foreskin, a fold of skin that covers the glans of the penis. This foreskin is often cut away by a doctor soon after the baby's birth, in an operation called a circumcision. In the Jewish and Muslim religions, the operation is performed in a religious rite. Once practiced for supposed hygienic reasons, the necessity of circumcision is increasingly being questioned: whether one has a foreskin or not will not affect sexual health or performance.

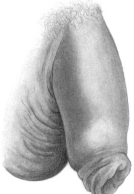
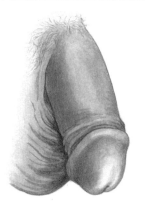

Uncircumcised penis   Circumcised penis

THE MALE REPRODUCTIVE ORGANS

The external organs are the penis and the testes. The testes hang in the scrotum, a pouch of skin behind the penis: the left usually hangs slightly lower than the right. During intercourse, semen is ejaculated from the penis into the woman's vagina to fertilize her eggs.

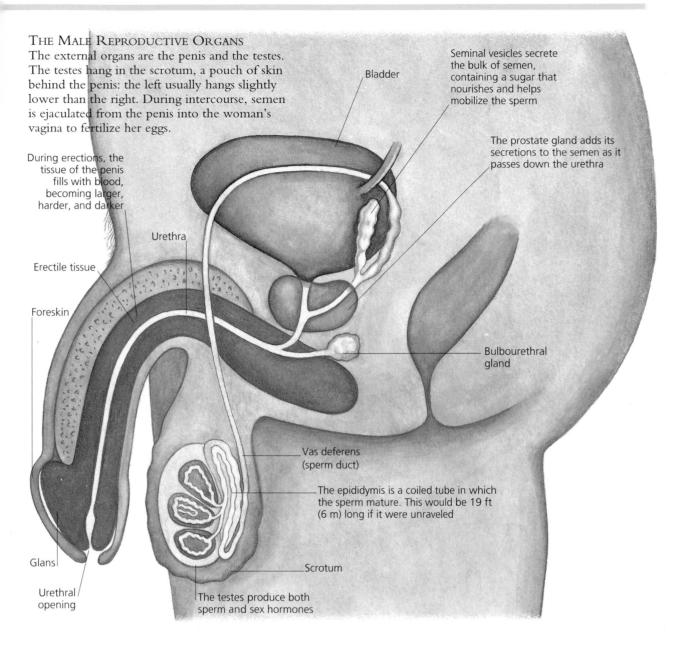

During erections, the tissue of the penis fills with blood, becoming larger, harder, and darker

Urethra

Erectile tissue

Foreskin

Glans

Urethral opening

Bladder

Seminal vesicles secrete the bulk of semen, containing a sugar that nourishes and helps mobilize the sperm

The prostate gland adds its secretions to the semen as it passes down the urethra

Bulbourethral gland

Vas deferens (sperm duct)

The epididymis is a coiled tube in which the sperm mature. This would be 19 ft (6 m) long if it were unraveled

Scrotum

The testes produce both sperm and sex hormones

QUESTIONS AND ANSWERS

Why do I seem to wake up with an erection every morning? Is this normal?
Paul, 14 years

This happens to many boys. Erections can occur in dreams, whether or not the dream is sexual, when it may result in a "wet dream" (*page 27*). Sometimes when you wake up with an erection it is just because your bladder is full.

Why do I keep having erections all the time, even when I'm not thinking about girls or anything?
Will, 14 years

Most boys have spontaneous erections, which are embarrassing if they happen at the wrong time or in the wrong place. They are caused by the raised levels of testosterone in the body and will stop as puberty passes. They do go away if you think about something else.

Is it true that wearing tight jeans can make a man infertile?
Joanna, 16 years

Anything that affects sperm production affects fertility. Tight jeans can raise the temperature of the scrotum, preventing sperm from developing properly. Sperm are produced all the time, however, so while wearing tight jeans may lower a man's fertility temporarily, it would not affect it in the future.

The body's sensuality

As the body matures, so does one's awareness of its sensitivity and sensuality. Discovering, exploring, and understanding its sensitivity can help one to enjoy sexual activity in the broadest sense: sexual enjoyment involves the whole body, not just the sex organs.

WHAT IS MASTURBATION?

Masturbation means touching or rubbing one's genitals or a partner's to give sexual pleasure, and usually to have an orgasm. Orgasm is a throbbing feeling that brings intense pleasure. For many people, masturbation is their first sexual experience. It is a harmless and natural way for people to enjoy their sexuality on their own. It relieves the tension that results from sexual urges and is a way to discover exciting sensations – knowledge that can be shared with a partner to show them how one likes to be aroused. Masturbation also helps the young appreciate that sexual pleasure is not the simple mechanical exercise so often represented in the media. Good sexual relations take time and consideration.

Some people find out about masturbation from brothers, sisters, or friends, while others discover it on their own. By the late teens, the majority of boys and girls will have masturbated. However, some people never feel a need to masturbate, and this is quite normal as well.

HOW PEOPLE MASTURBATE

There are no fixed ways to masturbate. Everyone does what pleases them. Many people daydream about a person they care about or pretend they are in a different place while they masturbate. Other people have sexual fantasies *(see page 28)*. All of this is completely normal.

Stimulation of the clitoris is the main way that girls experience orgasm. Girls generally rub and stroke around and over the clitoris with their fingers, moving faster and faster until they have an orgasm. As sexual excitement rises, the vagina becomes moist. Girls can have several orgasms, one after the other. Boys masturbate by stimulating the penis. Most boys hold their penis and move their hand up and down to stimulate it; some boys just rub the penis, increasing speed until they reach orgasm and semen is released, or ejaculated. The penis becomes limp after ejaculation.

Boys commonly experience arousal without masturbation while sleeping. A "wet dream" is the result of dreaming about

> **❝** *I just love having my ear lobes kissed. It drives me wild and makes me feel tingly inside.* **❞**
>
> Annette, 16 years

WHO MASTURBATES?

Surveys show that by their late teens, about 90 percent of boys masturbate. The numbers for girls vary from as low as 60 percent to as high as 80 percent. Social attitudes and education may account for these differences: sexual double standards and the discredited idea that women shouldn't enjoy sex might make girls feel more guilty about masturbating than boys, and make some girls less likely than others to masturbate.

something sexually exciting. As a result, the penis is aroused and ejaculates sperm, even though the boy is sleeping. A boy then wakes up because the semen is cold on his skin or wets his clothes. He might even be shocked because his dream was about a girl or boy whom he would not normally think about in a sexual way. Wet dreams are quite normal and are one sign that a person is becoming sexually mature, although not all boys have them. Boys may also experience spontaneous erections at unexpected times and even in public places.

Many girls also have dreams that make them sexually aroused, and sometimes they will have orgasms in their sleep. These are not really "wet" dreams though, because girls don't ejaculate.

> *I had my first orgasm while I was in the shower. Soaping myself down there felt really good, so I just kept going.*
> Martha, 15 years

> *I have really strange thoughts when I masturbate but I don't think I would ever do what I think about in real life.*
> Colin, 15 years

EROGENOUS ZONES

The body is covered with touch and pressure sensors that, when touched or stroked, can arouse a person sexually.

These are known as erogenous zones. The genitals are usually the most sensitive zones on the body.

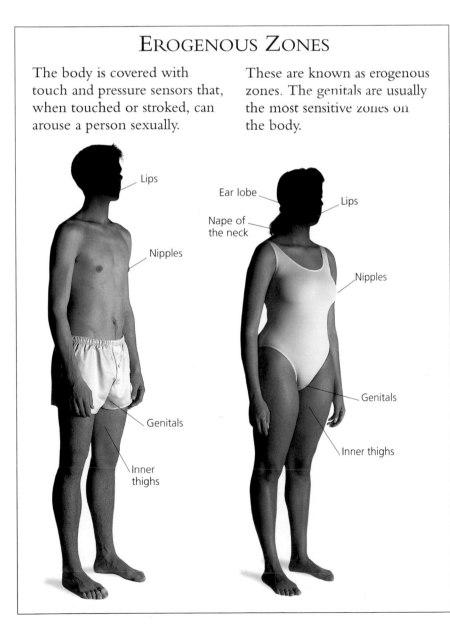

Lips

Ear lobe

Nape of the neck

Lips

Nipples

Nipples

Genitals

Genitals

Inner thighs

Inner thighs

❝ The first time I had a wet dream, I thought there was something wrong with me. When it happened to my younger brother, he was really embarrassed because he thought he'd wet the bed, and I had to explain it all to him. ❞
Brian, 18 years

GUILT AND MYTHS ABOUT MASTURBATION

Many people feel guilty about masturbating. Small children find natural pleasure in touching their genitals, only to be reprimanded by adults. This can lead to confusion and leave feelings of guilt and shame about touching themselves. These guilt feelings can conflict with their sexual urges when they reach puberty and, later, when they become sexually active.

Many parents will not talk to their children about masturbation, and some will tell them that masturbation is wrong. This is probably because of what their parents told them when they were young. Masturbation was once believed to cause poor health, loss of sight, paralysis, and madness, and boys and girls were punished for touching their genitals. Even today, some repeat the same fears and myths, but they are completely untrue and ought to be ignored.

SEXUAL FANTASIES

Most people have fantasies – or daydreams – at some time. Some might imagine that they are great athletes or singers or dream about what they will achieve. No one will ever know these thoughts, unless the person having them, reveals them. Sexual fantasies are the same. It is normal to have sexual fantasies during masturbation or at any other time. Some people worry because they fantasize about things they would never do in real life: some might imagine that they are having sex in public or with someone unexpected, or watching others have sex. How one thinks during sexual activity is a private, personal matter.

QUESTIONS AND ANSWERS

I'm in a football team. We've been told not to masturbate for 24 hours before games because it'll spoil our performance. Is this true?
Jon, 15 years

No. This is one of many masturbation myths. People once thought that masturbation would weaken your body, and, although totally false, the story lives on. What you do with your body is your own business and nobody else's.

Do older people still masturbate if they're married or living together?
Terri, 15 years

Many people do. They may do it on their own, or with – or to – their partner.

If I don't have sex or anything, will all the sperm build up in my balls and make them burst?
Leroy, 14 years

No: unused sperm are stored for a while until they get old, and then they are reabsorbed into your body and replaced.

I heard that masturbation changes how the vulva looks. Will my doctor be able to tell that I do it?
Thea, 17 years

No. Masturbation does not change your genitals, so nobody can tell. But don't worry if you ever need to tell your doctor that you masturbate (if you have some sexual problem, for instance): they know that it is normal.

RELATIONSHIPS AND EMOTIONS

Changing feelings ■ *Friends* ■
Social life ■ *Looking at others* ■
Starting a relationship ■
Sexual preference ■ *Emotional decisions* ■

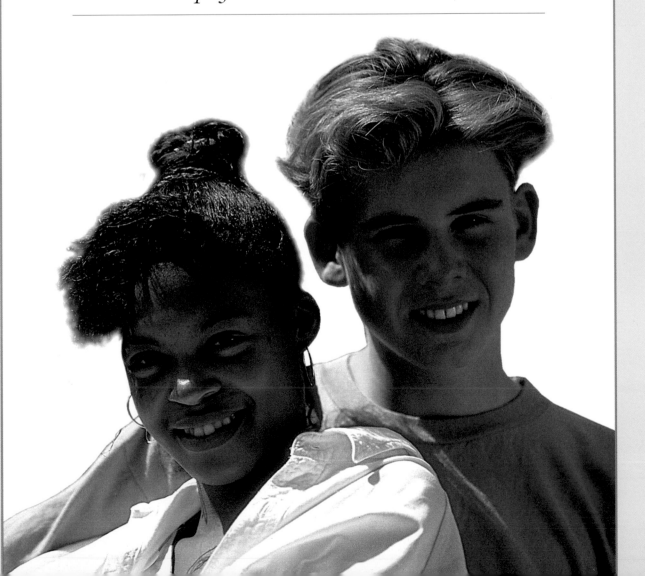

Changing feelings

In adolescence, feelings are often changing as fast as the body. The young person feels things more deeply and becomes more emotional. This is a time when a person may be happy one day, miserable or irritable the next. This is a tumultuous time and an exciting one.

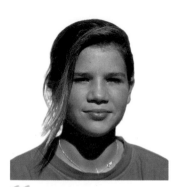

When I look at myself in the mirror, I hate myself. I'm too fat and my hair is all wrong. When I go out, I feel like everyone is looking at me.

Marisa, 16 years

FEELING SELF-CONSCIOUS

The body is changing so rapidly that it may seem that everything – hair, shape, and skin – is wrong. It is common for a young person to feel awkward and self-conscious, or worried about being attractive. Remember, everyone has their good points physically, whether a smile, freckles, shining eyes, or dimples in their cheeks. And we all know that it isn't just looks that makes people attractive; a sense of humor and friendliness, for example, are just as important.

CHANGING RELATIONSHIPS WITH FRIENDS

Relationships become more intense during adolescence. Friends in general become more important: friendships made in adolescence last longer than those made during childhood, and when a friendship does break up, as it probably will, it can be especially painful.

Some will develop a close, best friend now, or a group of friends they see all the time. It often feels more comfortable to form friendships as part of a group at first; a one-to-one relationship can then develop naturally.

INDEPENDENCE AND CONFLICT

Adolescents' relationships with their families will probably change dramatically during these years. Teens may find there are some topics they don't want to discuss with their parents or siblings – not because they are doing anything wrong, but simply because they are trying to develop their own independence. Often these feelings of independence lead to conflict.

Some may feel that their parents expect too much of them, or that they want them just like they are. Those who have been brought up with certain beliefs and attitudes may begin to question them and be interested in finding out about others. This can lead to conflict in families. It is not always easy for parents to accept their children's different views and attitudes. It is important to discuss such issues openly with parents as well as friends to avoid unnecessary, possibly painful, conflicts.

UNDERSTANDING PARENTS' FEELINGS

Sex is often an uncomfortable subject between parents and children. Some parents find it difficult to accept that their child is growing up sexually. No matter what their own experience was when they were teens, they will probably feel differently when it comes to their child. Some teens find that their parents read sex and danger into every situation, or refuse to accept their child's sexuality, or change the subject whenever sex is mentioned. Some teens might find themselves educating their parents; there are free pamphlets available from various agencies and counseling centers that give advice to children and parents.

It's natural for a loving parent to worry, especially when their child starts to go out on his or her own. Discussing concerns openly and trying to see things from a parent's point of view can help keep the lines of communication open.

SEXUAL THOUGHTS AND FEELINGS

Sometimes sexual feelings may be so strong that they make it hard to think about anything else. These feelings need someone to focus on, and this can be almost anyone. It is very common for an adolescent to have a crush on a teacher or an unattainable rock star, even though realistically there is no hope of forming a real relationship. However strong such feelings are, that is all they are. They don't necessarily mean that one is emotionally ready to start a sexual relationship yet. Learning not to respond to every physical urge is just as important a part of growing up as learning how to save money or eating a well-balanced diet and not just sweets.

> *I know I ought not to worry and nag, but unless she's okay, I worry and I can't sleep. Now she telephones if she is coming home late, and then I can relax.*
>
> Derek, father

QUESTIONS AND ANSWERS

I'm writing to this girl I met on vacation. My parents are always asking me about her. They seem to think they have a right to know everything. Do they?
Mike, 15 years

It sounds as though your parents can't accept that your emotional life is private, perhaps because they are afraid you may be hurt and they want to protect you. However, your feelings are your own and very personal – you do not have to share them with anyone else unless you want to. Let your parents know gently that you want some privacy.

Sometimes I feel like bursting into tears – for no reason at all, really. My mother always says I'm just in one of my moods and tells me to snap out of it. But how am I supposed to do that?
Sarah, 14 years

You can't snap out of it just like that. But you will feel better if you tell someone how you feel: talking to a friend may help you see things differently. Activity helps these moods too, the more physical the better. Remember that when you are feeling low, everything looks bleak, and that this is just a passing mood.

Friends

Childhood friendships don't always last. It's during junior high and high school that many friendships that will last throughout life will be made. Friendships made during adolescence can include peers as well as teachers or other older role models.

BEING A GOOD FRIEND

Being part of a group of friends gives one a sense of belonging as well as self-confidence. If your friends like you, you feel good about yourself. This can work both ways: if you feel good about yourself, people will be comfortable with you. Those who are unkind, too critical, or talk only about themselves won't be much in demand as friends.

Friends will probably come from among classmates at school, or be people with similar interests, or neighbors. The most popular people don't necessarily make the best friends. People who seem different from you in some way may pleasantly surprise you once you get to know one another.

A good friend is often the person with whom you share all the ups and downs of becoming an adult, exchanging the secrets you wouldn't dream of discussing with your parents.

RESISTING PRESSURE FROM FRIENDS

Most young people want to be like their friends, dress like them, look like them, go where they go, and do what they do. Most of all, they value the opinion of their friends, and being part of a group and all the strengths and security it offers. Sometimes it can be hard to resist when your friends try to persuade you to do something you don't feel like doing, such as smoking, drinking, trying drugs, or skipping school. Experimentation is part of growing up, but it's up to you to decide when and if you want to experiment. You may also be under pressure to have sex before you feel ready for it.

Whenever you are under this kind of pressure, the most important thing to remember is that you don't have to lose good friends over it. Friends who drop you if you don't do everything they do are not worth having in the long run: good friends will respect you if you are your own person, and not just a mirror of them. This can take real courage, though, because it isn't comfortable to be left out. You don't have to be critical, you can just say "That doesn't feel right for me." The more sure of yourself you sound, the less pressure there is likely to be.

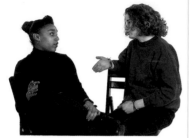

My best friend and I always talk for hours every day, and we talk about everything. If anything's wrong, we can always cheer each other up.

Amy, 12 years

BEATING SHYNESS

It's hard to stop being shy, but you can learn to act as if you're not.

■ Practice playing the part of a nonshy person: it will eventually become natural.
■ Look at the person you are talking to. If you look past them or down at your feet, you will look bored.
■ Try to forget about yourself. Concentrate on other people and what's going on around you.
■ Pretend that the other person is shy, and try to put them at their ease.
■ If you get tongue-tied, at least ask a question or make a comment, even if "great" is all you say.

STARTING TO DATE

Most of your closest friends will probably be of your own sex. You might be interested in the opposite sex, think about them, and talk about them with your friends, but you may not feel quite as comfortable with them as you do with your own sex.

Going around in a mixed group of friends is often the easiest way to get to know one another. Couples may pair off within the group, but you might find yourself dating just to prove that you can, rather than because you really enjoy someone's company. These first relationships may not last very long, but they do help you experience closer relationships based on sexual attraction. By the time you're 17 or 18, you may be much better able to make more serious relationships.

FEELING LEFT OUT

Making and keeping friends is not always easy. You may feel as if you are the odd one out, that everyone else is having a great time, and that you are the only one who is feeling insecure and shy. But these are very common feelings, shared by even apparently confident people.

If you find it hard to make friends, remember that they don't just fall into your lap. Everyone has to work to make friends, and if you always wait around for others to make the first move, you may have to wait a long time. You could also choose a more active route – join a youth club, take up a hobby, or go out for a sport at school.

There's a boy in our class who has a really rough time because his mother buys him these awful clothes. I feel sorry for him, but I'm afraid that if I talk to him, I'll get picked on too.

Kevin, 13 years

FRIENDSHIP
Shared interests provide the basis for friendship – these might include an interest in music, movies, fashion, art, or sports.

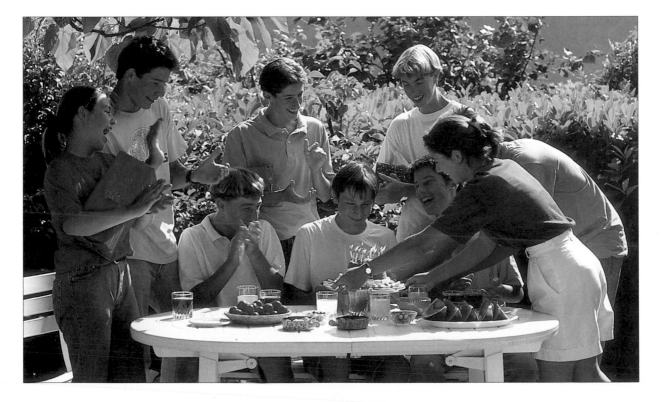

Social life

It is natural as you grow up that you'll want to spend more time with your own friends. Going places and doing things with friends who are interested in the same sorts of things is the start of an exciting new phase and time of discovery in your social life.

Freedom to be yourself

Sometimes you may feel that you are quite a different person with your friends than you are at home. Parents may have a strong idea what their child is like and find it difficult to accept their child's increasing sense of self-sufficiency and desire for independence. Your friends, like you, are also growing, changing, and experimenting and so it is natural to feel more comfortable with them. Sometimes this can cause friction at home because your parents may not approve of the way they see you are changing.

Parents and friends

If your parents dislike or disapprove of your friends, it is probably because they don't know them. They may have formed an impression based solely on the way your friends look or dress. It may help if you use your home as a base for your social life for a while; when your parents get to know your friends better they may understand why you like them. If they refuse to accept these friendships, and you truly value your friends, you are left with the difficult choice of giving up your friends, or confronting your parents and asking them to trust you.

Smoking and drinking

Alcohol, cigarettes, and drugs are substances teens are inevitably exposed to, and are all dangerous when abused. Alcohol and drugs both lower inhibitions and can lead people to behave less cautiously than

All my friends smoke, but I just coughed and felt horrible. It's too expensive anyway.
Clare, 16 years

Your Closest Friends
As adolescence progresses, groups of boys and girls mix more, even though your closest friends may still be your own sex.

usual or than they would choose to, if not under their influence. Many unprotected sexual experiences as well as traffic accidents happen as the result of being temporarily out of control.

The dangers of alcohol abuse as well as drug abuse among teens should not be underestimated. Teens are by nature risk takers, but it is important that they learn what their own bodies can safely tolerate and that they learn to set limits. Girls in particular need to know that in general their tolerance level for alcohol is lower than that of boys. Many boys and girls have, when drunk, done things sexually that they have later regretted.

Tobacco is another drug that carries significant health risks. Although it may seem like fun to experiment with smoking cigarettes, their connection to lung cancer and other health problems has been clearly established. Being fully informed about any substance one wants to try is always a good idea, and may help a young person decide what to try and how much.

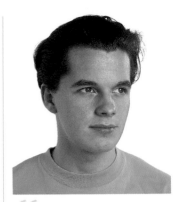

" My parents are so concerned about the furniture, I couldn't ask my friends home. Something would get broken. It's better to hang out at the mall or in the park. "
Josh, 17 years

QUESTIONS AND ANSWERS

Why is it that I only have two or three drinks and I start feeling drunk very quickly?
Naomi, 16 years

Girls shouldn't try to keep pace with boys. With the same amount of alcohol in the bloodstream, girls become drunk much more quickly because their bodies contain less water than boy's. Have a meal or snack before you drink. You get drunk more quickly if your stomach is empty. Have some water or soft drinks first to quench your thirst. Learn to say no and switch to soft drinks when you've had enough. This way you will avoid doing something you will later regret.

What is sensible drinking?
Oliver, 17 years

It is sensible to limit your alcohol intake to two drinks on the weekend. Drinking beer or alcohol daily can be a sign of dependence. Binge drinking is especially dangerous, and can be fatal. Don't take lifts from anyone you know who has been drinking, and never drive yourself if you have been drinking.

Why is my boyfriend so aggressive when he drinks?
Anna, 16 years

Alcohol changes behavior. Often people don't realize how much until friends tell them the next day what they did while they were drunk. Tell your boyfriend that you don't like the side of his character that shows itself when he drinks too much.

It's really hard to avoid drugs at the parties I go to. What should I do about this?
Emily, 16 years

You should never be afraid to say no if you don't want to use drugs. If some of your friends are experimenting with drugs, you may be tempted to experiment yourself. You have to make up your mind if the risks are worth taking. If you do experiment, find out all you can about the drug first so that you know what the dangers are. Ecstasy, for example, can cause dangerous dehydration and other serious problems. Never experiment on your own; make sure you are with people you know and trust.

" I got pregnant because I was drunk, and I didn't even ask if he used a condom. I really don't remember much. "
Annette, 16 years

Looking at others

Everyone has expectations of themselves and of others, and these may not always be realistic or fair. Sometimes they are based on stereotypes that can affect the way we see the world. Real people, however, don't conform to such patterns.

WHAT IS A STEREOTYPE?

Stereotypes are generalizations about groups of people – perhaps a social class or ethnic group – and they are often the root cause of prejudice. Stereotypes are inaccurate and unfair. They encourage you to think of someone as a type because of their gender or color or appearance, for example, rather than as an individual.

REJECTING SOME OLD IDEAS

In the last 30 years social attitudes have changed in many ways. These changes have made it easier for both men and women to break out of many of their traditional roles if they want to – girls become doctors, women have successful careers, boys experiment with clothes and take on more domestic roles.

Old rules about sexual relationships need not apply today. There's no good reason, for example, why a girl shouldn't ask

The first thing dad said when I told him I didn't want to play football was "That's ridiculous, I was a great athlete and so are you." He just couldn't believe I wanted to study art.
Mark, 18 years

HAPPY FAMILIES

Today in the United States, two out of every three marriages end in divorce. Living with a stepparent or relating to divorced parents creates added pressures for an adolescent. However, chances are there are many others who share your concerns and who can help you realize your family is actually normal by today's standards.

QUESTIONS AND ANSWERS

My parents have told me that they are separating and probably getting a divorce. What can I do?
Katrina, 14 years

If your parents are divorcing, try to understand that they have decided to be honest by separating instead of staying together and being unhappy. If the atmosphere at home has been very bad, the divorce may even be a relief to you. But if they are so preoccupied with their problems that they are unaware of your anxieties and possible guilt feelings, talk to your brothers and sisters or a close friend. You can give real comfort to each other in this difficult situation. If you are really distressed and have no one to turn to, there are telephone helplines with counselors who can give you advice (*see pages 92-93*).

My friend picks on me about not having a dad. I want to tell him to shut up. What should I say?
David, 15 years

The two-parent, married, heterosexual couple is widely regarded as "normal," although it is far from being the only model. Being a good parent need not have anything to do with being married or single, or straight or gay. Conventional married couples don't necessarily make good parents – successful parenting depends on the ability of the people involved to have a loving and caring relationship with their children. Tell your friend you feel happy with your parent, and that he should stop looking at people as stereotypes but as individuals. Perhaps he isn't such a good friend!

a boy out. The best relationships are based on honesty and equality and have no set roles. Sometimes one of you will want to be cuddled and cared for, sometimes the other; sometimes one person will have definite ideas about where to go or what to do. You don't have to fit in with someone else's idea of how you ought to behave.

TREATING GIRLS DIFFERENTLY

There is one persistent stereotype that doesn't seem to go away. A boy who boasts about his sexual exploits and has many different sexual partners is regarded as a real man, while a girl who sleeps with a number of different boys is sometimes branded as loose and easy. The message is that girls shouldn't have any sexual desires, or that they shouldn't do anything about them. This is unequal treatment and untrue. Both boys and girls have sexual desires – the real issue for both is learning when and when not to respond to those desires, and how to act intelligently and with caution to avoid doing something they may later regret.

❝I'm much better at math and science than most of the boys in our class, but I feel I have to keep quiet.❞

Sue, 14 years

ENRICHING EXPERIENCE
If you live in a multicultural area, you will probably mix with people whose backgrounds are very different from your own.

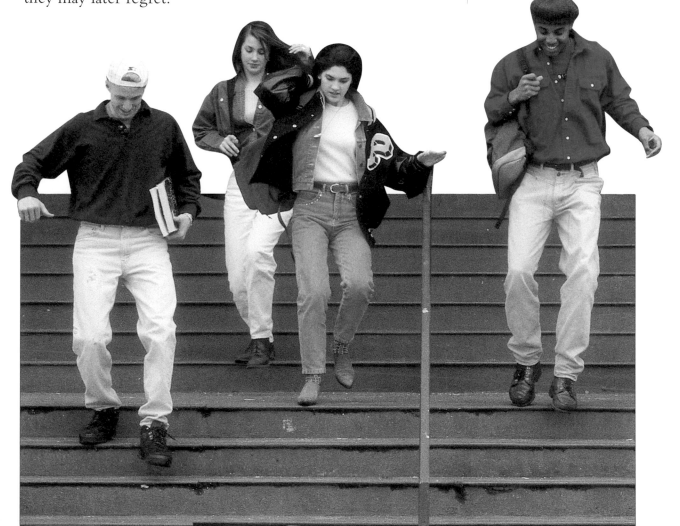

Starting a relationship

People may know instinctively that they want to get to know someone better. Making the first move is a gamble because there is the chance of being turned down. But, without trying, nothing can happen, so why not try?

THE PERFECT PARTNER

Most people think they have some idea of their ideal type. Quite often, however, they find themselves falling for someone totally different, who they were not initially attracted to at all. Friendship, good conversation, a sense of humor, liking the same music, or an interest in sports could all be the basis of an attraction to a particular person.

SHOWING AND EXPRESSING FEELINGS

You can show that you like someone by seeking out their company, looking into their eyes a bit more than usual when you talk, or touching them casually – a hand on their arm to attract their attention, for example. If someone shows this kind of interest in you, it's up to you how you respond. If you feel the same, you can smile back, hold their gaze, and not move away. If you want to discourage their advances, you can be a bit aloof without being rude, giving them a cue to back off.

Body language works, up to a point, but it is more honest to say what you feel. Once you are over the "getting-to-know-you" stage, misunderstandings can be avoided if you can tell each other, as well as show each other, how you feel.

> *I knew he liked me, but he just wouldn't say anything. So I went and sat beside him at lunch and got talking, and after that everything was fine.*
>
> Jenny, 15 years

ATTRACTION

It's no accident that lovers tend to gaze into one another's eyes. The pupil in the eye widens when we look at something that interests or attracts us. Most of us agree on what makes a "beautiful" face, but differ on what we find sexually attractive. Statistically, physical appearance matters more to men, while women are usually attracted by a man's intelligence and sense of humor rather than by his looks.

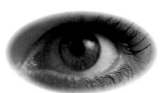
Pupils narrow

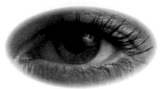
Pupils widen

Of course, you probably won't like everyone who likes you, so you may have to tell someone you're not interested. If someone you aren't really interested in approaches you, remember that it took courage for them to ask you out. It is kinder to be polite if you're not interested than cruelly to reject someone.

COMING ON STRONG

Trying to get too close to someone too soon is usually a big mistake. You can't force someone to like you. Look for cues that you are moving too fast, and slow down. If you draw attention to yourself, tell too many jokes, or praise people profusely because you want them to like you, you will start to look desperate and drive the person away.

At the start of a relationship, it is often hard not to try to take over the other person completely. But relationships need time to grow. Resist the temptation to demand that your boy or girlfriend be with you all the time.

THREE'S A CROWD

It can happen to anyone: you like someone a friend of yours is going out with. What should you do? You could show that you're interested, but the chances are that you will lose your friend this way. You could also ask your friend how serious the relationship is. You have to decide which means most to you – your friendship or a possible future relationship. It can be just as difficult to find that you are interested in a friend of the person you're going out with. Think carefully before you make any advance. Of the three of you, at least one will get hurt, and it could be you.

GOOD RELATIONSHIPS

Falling in love can be thrilling. Your heart pounds, and there are butterflies in your stomach, and you'll long to be together every moment and think about each other compulsively. A good relationship is one that increases the self-esteem and personal happiness of both people involved. It is also one that is based on mutual respect, good communication, and trust. Being good friends is vital in a relationship.

A couple may enjoy going out and socializing with others; or may just be happy being alone together. Being in a relationship gives one the opportunity to listen to someone else's views intently and to learn to resolve differences. It is not always easy to tell the short-term infatuation from the relationship that will last. Everyone is bound to make a few mistakes as they are growing up. Most, in fact, look back later and wonder what they ever saw in that person who once seemed to be the most important person in their life.

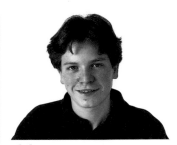

I didn't ask this girl out for ages – I was afraid she'd turn me down or laugh. She said yes, though, and she said she'd been waiting for me to say something. I had no idea!

Keith, 15 years

I went out with this girl for a few weeks, thinking this is it! Then suddenly I realized I didn't want to see her any more – she looks fantastic, but she's a bit boring when you get to know her.

Sean, 16 years

Sexual preference

Part of growing up is discovering what your main sexual preferences are. It is very common for teens to be confused about the range of strong sexual feelings they experience. Many worry if they find themselves attracted to their own sex or to both sexes.

EXPRESSING YOUR SEXUALITY

By a very early age our gender identity as a boy or girl is established. What happens later in life in terms of how we experience our sexuality – how we think, feel, and act as a male or female – involves value judgments and choice. Few people go through life without ever having felt attracted to someone of their own sex. Teenagers often have passionate sexual feelings for a friend or a teacher. Girls are just as likely as boys to have homosexual feelings. But feelings and fantasies are not necessarily an indication of what will ultimately be one's sexual preference. For many, this is a practice stage of sexual development, while some will continue to be attracted by their own sex at some times in their lives, and by the opposite sex at others. As one grows to adulthood, it is usual for a steady preference for one sex or the other to emerge, although there are people who will be bisexual.

WHAT CAUSES THESE FEELINGS?

Nobody knows exactly why some people are attracted to their own sex and others to the opposite sex. Some believe sexual preference is learned behavior, while others believe heredity, environment and upbringing play a part. During adolescence, when so much is changing, a passing homosexual infatuation does not mean one will as an adult have a preference for same-sex relationships. It is wise not to overreact to early fleeting stirrings of homosexual attraction.

COMING TO TERMS WITH HOMOSEXUALITY

Because society treats heterosexuality as the norm, young people who experience homosexual feelings regularly may be uncomfortable in talking about them. There is no denying that there is prejudice against homosexuals. Those who are attracted to their own sex will be tempted to keep quiet about it when they hear their classmates use "gay" as a term of abuse. An older teenager who has experienced homosexual feelings for

I think my parents hoped they could cure me of being gay, and that it was all just in my imagination.

Mark, 18 years

FINDING OUT
Once you've accepted your own feelings, you'll discover that there are plenty of other people who feel like you do.

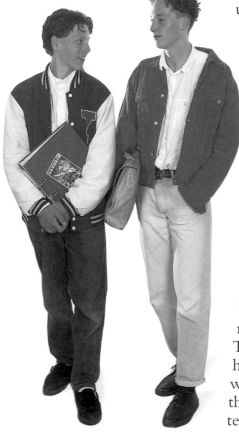

years and who has identified himself or herself as a homosexual will inevitably encounter problems created by other people's prejudice and intolerance. Knowing this, some gay and lesbian people choose to try to ignore their feelings or disguise their sexuality. This can cause a great deal of unhappiness. Those who are sure of their feelings may feel more comfortable telling the truth to those who matter most to them. A consolation is that society in general is becoming more accepting of homosexuality.

INFORMING PARENTS

One hard decision to make for anyone who knows they are gay or lesbian is whether to tell their parents. Understandably, unsuspecting parents may be upset at first and will almost certainly need time to get used to the idea. Many people think that there is only one way to live and be happy and that is their way. Some parents may have strong religious convictions, and some may think that unless their child has a conventional marriage with children, they won't be happy. And whatever their own feelings, they know also that gays and lesbians are often treated unfairly. They'll also be worried about AIDS.

However, the advantages of telling one's parents and not having to keep a very important part of one's life secret are enormous. It is quite possible that some parents may have guessed, anyway. Loving parents can eventually accept that their child is gay or lesbian.

Some will want a trial run before they tell their parents. A close family friend might be a good person to tell first. They can act as a support when broaching the subject with parents. A close friend who can be trusted and who will listen and be sympathetic is also a vital source of support. Teens can also seek a counselor or trusted teacher or seek out a gay and lesbian organization (*see pages 92-93*) for peer group counseling.

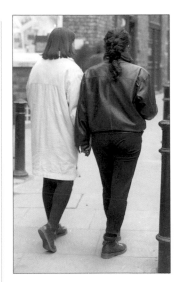

BEING TOGETHER
A loving relationship with someone they care about is what most people want, whether they are gay, lesbian, or straight.

❝ When I called the hotline I realized that she was the first lesbian person I had knowingly talked to. It was comforting. ❞

Sue, 16 years

QUESTIONS AND ANSWERS

What is it that gay and lesbian people do?
Sean, 16 years

Gay and lesbians lead normal lives in which they experience the same sexual and emotional feelings as heterosexuals. They want to be near one another, kiss, and make love like heterosexual people. They can show their sexual feelings through sexual activity and loving and caring companionship.

I usually dream about boys, but last night I dreamt I was kissing my girlfriend. Am I a lesbian?
Jane, 15 years

Everyone fantasizes and dreams about sex. Your dream shows that you love your friend, but it does not mean that you are a lesbian. Such dreams are completely normal.

THE LAW

Every state has laws about sexual intercourse. Because the law in many states makes it illegal for a girl under 16 to have intercourse, 16 has been called "the age of consent." For boys there is no legal age of consent for heterosexual sex, but there are laws about homosexual activity - some states have laws making certain homosexual acts illegal for anyone.

Emotional decisions

Being in love is wonderful. It brings with it many confused emotions and exciting sensations, like having chills run up your spine when you hear that special person's voice on the phone. It takes time to learn how to handle the extreme feelings of the teenage years.

MAKING IT WORK

In the first flush of love, you may think your partner is perfect, but after this infatuation passes, you begin to see each other as real people. If there's nothing much between you but sexual attraction, you may soon become bored and easily irritated with one another. Infatuation and a lasting relationship are not the same thing.

Learning how to handle a relationship takes work, and this is one reason why first relationships might be brief. This can be shattering, and rejection can be painful. But you do learn more with each relationship. What you get from a relationship is, more or less, what you put into it.

THINKING OF OTHERS

When you are in a relationship, you'll find yourself thinking about your partner a lot of the time. If their attitude toward you seems to change, don't take this too personally. Your partner may have moods that have nothing to do with you, so ask them what's wrong, instead of becoming offended and sulking. Learning to communicate in a relationship is very important. This means being able to express what you want, as well as finding out about your partner's needs.

BEING OUT OF STEP

Boys and girls tend to be out of step with one another in their teens. Emotionally, girls usually grow up more quickly than boys; a boy of 15 can seem very childish to a girl of the same age. As a result, some girls are likely to be interested in more mature boys. Because of this, girls often come under pressure to have sex earlier than they might want to, especially if they go out with older boys or men.

HOW FAR SHOULD YOU GO?

Movies, magazines, and books often seem to suggest that there's only one road for a relationship to go down, and it ends in bed. This is not the case in real life. Each person is an individual and each must decide how far to go and when to

---

We really love each other, but I feel I've met the right person at the wrong time. I wish I could just put the whole thing on ice for five years.

Anna, 16 years

HOW TO SAY NO

Saying no when you are confronted with a difficult social or sexual situation takes practice.

■ Body language gives the other person the hint quite quickly. Straighten up and move back, keeping some distance between you so that you can get your thoughts clear.

■ Practice saying no in situations where it is justified – if your little brother or sister is being unreasonably demanding, or if someone wants to borrow a pen that you need, too.

■ Don't give in to bullying by being made to feel different. Recognize that coercion can be subtle. For example, someone might say: "If you don't have sex, you'll be the only virgin in your group."

stop. Some may not want a sexual relationship yet, or not with this person. Some have strong religious, cultural, and personal views about sex outside marriage and should not be afraid to uphold their views. And, in this time, when it is easy to contract a sexually transmitted disease, many teens are choosing to take it very slow. No one ever died from not having sex.

You'll meet plenty of people whom you like, even love, but want nothing more than a kiss or a hug from, and who may feel the same about you. It is possible to have a loving and caring relationship without sex. The most important thing is to make clear what *you* want, and to make your own choices, especially if you think that the other person might have something else in mind. If you don't know what you want, say so and be assertive. You have a right to make up your own mind without being pressured. No one should force you into having full penetrative sex that you don't want or don't feel ready for.

THE RIGHT TIME AND THE RIGHT PERSON

When you have reached the age of consent – and this differs from state to state and country to country – you can have sexual intercourse legally. This doesn't mean it's compulsory, and it is usually too early for most people. While a 16-year-old, for example, is physically old enough to have sexual intercourse and to have a baby, few 16-year-olds are emotionally mature enough to deal with the commitments and responsibilities involved in a lasting sexual relationship.

There are no prizes for starting early; this is one of the hardest areas to be truthful about when your friends start and you don't want to be left out. Don't always believe what you hear – statistics show that by the age of 17 just under half of all boys and about a third of girls will have had sexual intercourse – so someone isn't telling the truth if you hear "Everybody but you is having sex." If you have doubts, or feel you need more advice and guidance (*see pages 92-93*), then you are probably not ready to have sex just yet. Being pressured to have sex can make it difficult to reach your own decision.

BREAKING UP

Breaking up can be much worse if you don't know why it happens. If the person you want to be with won't answer the phone or letters, you may know that it is over, but if they don't talk to you, you might just keep hoping. It is always kinder to be honest and tell someone when a relationship is over.

WHEN TO SAY NO

If you are thinking of having sex for any of the following reasons, it is better to say no.
■ To prove you love someone or as proof of their love.
■ To prove you can (everyone can!)
■ To satisfy your curiosity.
■ Because you're afraid that you will lose your boyfriend or girlfriend if you don't.
■ Because you've been talked into it.
■ Because you are drunk or high on drugs.
■ Because the other person expects it.

Mom started telling me to go on the pill when she saw I was getting serious with Tony. I know she meant well, but I can make up my own mind about when I want to sleep with someone.
Jill, 17 years

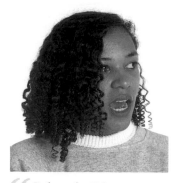

I thought I'd never get over it. Then my friend persuaded me to go out with her, and I met Alan. We are so happy together! I never thought I'd feel like this again.
Melanie, 16 years

Anyone determined to have sex should make sure it is planned and protected (*see page 54*). Statistics show that early sexual experiences are often spontaneous and as a result unprotected. One's first sexual experience can be fantastic or a real disappointment – even if it is with the right person at the right time and in the right place. This first experience is seen as a rite of passage, and an important point in one's life – don't waste it with the wrong person at the wrong time.

WHEN FEELINGS CHANGE

Relationships don't stand still. One person might want to get more serious, while the other still wants to see other people. Part of maturing is learning what to do as a relationship evolves. Some might find it possible to negotiate a way to go on with a relationship like this, while others might find it too painful.

It hurts to discover that the other person doesn't feel as deeply as you do, and it can be just as hard to find that you don't love someone as much as you hoped you might. It takes courage to end things when you still care for the other person, but it might be necessary. Having sex within this relationship won't save it either, nor will it stop your partner from moving on.

LETTING SOMEONE DOWN GENTLY

It's always painful for both people involved when a relationship breaks up. Teenagers often believe that they'll never be happy again, but with time, feelings change. Talking with friends can help. A definite good-bye may hurt, but everything will be easier once a person accepts that the relationship is over. Then it is possible to go forward, stronger and wiser for the experience.

THE AGE OF CONSENT

State laws regarding sexual intercourse vary. Because the law in many states makes it illegal for a girl under 16 to have intercourse, 16 has been called the "age of consent." For boys, there is no legal age of consent for heterosexual sex, but there are laws about homosexual activity (*see page 41*).

QUESTIONS AND ANSWERS

My friends all keep telling me to keep away from this girl I like at school, because she treated her last boyfriend really badly. But can't things be different for us?
Martin, 16 years

Seeing how people have behaved in other relationships is a clue to their behavior but it doesn't tell the whole story. Perhaps you are hearing a biased account and the truth is very different. Hurt pride can cause people to be spiteful and tell lies. Spend some time getting to know the girl and find out for yourself what she is like.

My boyfriend and I have been together for six months and we get along really well together, but we don't have a lot in common. Does this matter?
Kristy, 16 years

You don't have to call the whole thing off because you don't share a passion for all the same things. Similar personalities, backgrounds, or interests are all pluses in any relationship, but although they help, they aren't essential. As long as you enjoy each other's company, there isn't a problem; it is probably the differences that attract you to one another.

WHAT HAPPENS DURING SEX

- Sexual intercourse
- The first time
- Enjoying sex
- Dealing with difficulties

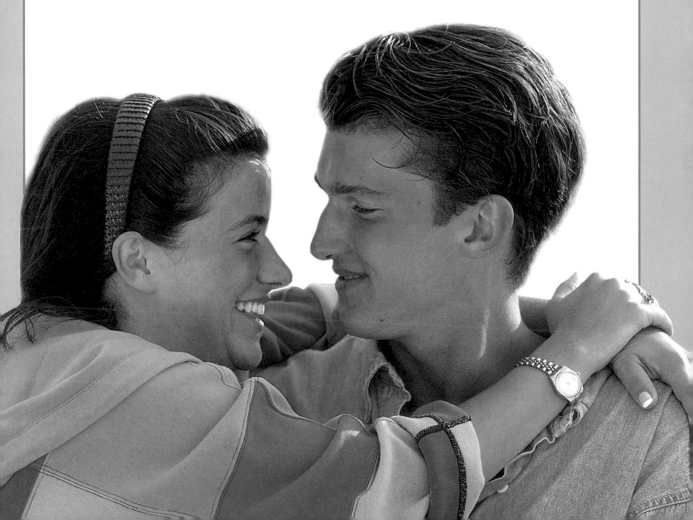

Sexual intercourse

Sexual intercourse, or making love, is an intimate form of contact between two people. Its biological function is to enable a woman to become pregnant, but when couples have sex they mostly do so simply because they enjoy it.

FOREPLAY AND AROUSAL

A couple arouse one another by holding, caressing, and kissing: this is called foreplay. They can stroke or kiss the sensitive areas of one another's bodies – the stomach, inner thighs, buttocks, nipples, and around the highly sensitive genitals. The smell and taste of a partner's skin and genitals enhance sexual excitement.

During foreplay, the body's senses are stimulated, sending messages to the brain, which, in turn, sends messages to the genitals and other parts of the body, preparing them for sex and increasing excitement. Many men and some women can be sexually aroused by the sight of their partner's body and the thought of sex.

WHAT HAPPENS WHEN SOMEONE IS AROUSED

When people are aroused, their heart and breathing rates increase, and their bodies feel super-sensitive. Both sexes also experience changes in their genitals. Arousal increases blood flow into the penis, causing it to extend, darken, and become erect. As the man becomes more excited, his penis reaches its

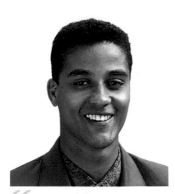

We spend more time on foreplay before sex than we used to, and we both have better orgasms – they're more intense.

Nick, 18 years

I get really hot during sex, and my heart pounds. It's better exercise than working out!

Leonie, 17 years

QUESTIONS AND ANSWERS

My boyfriend says if I don't have sex with him it means I don't love him. But I don't feel ready, what can I do?
Zoë, 16 years

Follow your instincts. When you are ready, you will know. If he respects you, he will stop asking.

How long should you spend on foreplay before having sex?
Barry, 17 years

Foreplay should be long enough for both partners to become excited enough to enjoy intercourse. Men

sometimes forget that women can take longer to become aroused than men.

A friend told me sex isn't complete without intercourse. But can't you have orgasms in other ways?
Darryl, 17 years

Sex needn't mean intercourse. Some couples regularly have sex without intercourse (see page 58), arousing each other in other ways, and the orgasms they have are just as satisfying. This is also a way of practicing safer sex.

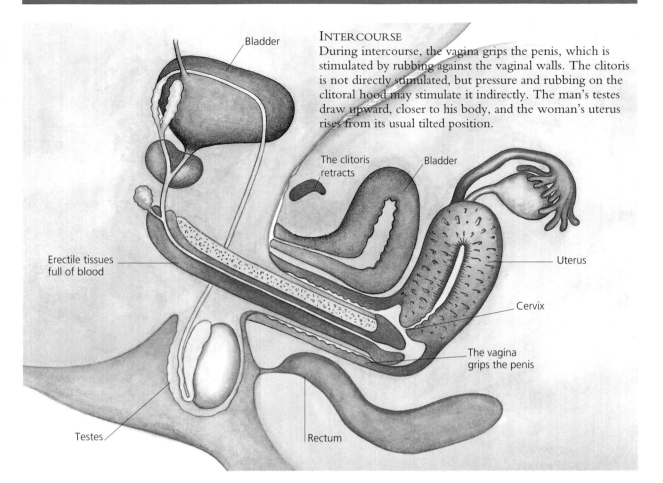

Bladder

INTERCOURSE

During intercourse, the vagina grips the penis, which is stimulated by rubbing against the vaginal walls. The clitoris is not directly stimulated, but pressure and rubbing on the clitoral hood may stimulate it indirectly. The man's testes draw upward, closer to his body, and the woman's uterus rises from its usual tilted position.

The clitoris retracts

Bladder

Erectile tissues full of blood

Uterus

Cervix

The vagina grips the penis

Testes

Rectum

maximum length and thickness. When a woman is aroused, the blood flow to her vulva and vagina increases. Her vagina becomes lubricated with mucus and its inner part expands. Her clitoris and her nipples become erect and more sensitive. As she grows more excited, her clitoris retracts, and her vaginal lips become bigger and darker.

INTERCOURSE AND ORGASM

When both partners are aroused, they may both feel ready for penetration (when the man's penis enters the vagina), though there are other ways of reaching orgasm (*see page 51*) without penetration. Orgasm is experienced by both sexes as a series of deep and pleasurable waves that spread throughout the whole body. Men and women don't necessarily reach orgasm in the same way and at the same time. The man often experiences orgasm as he ejaculates. A woman may not have an orgasm unless the clitoris is directly stimulated. Girls don't always find early experiences of sex orgasmic for this reason. Gradually man and women learn what gives them pleasure so they can let their partner know what they want. After ejaculation, the penis becomes limp and the man's excitement disappears. The woman's body returns to normal more gradually.

> *When my boyfriend comes, he sort of stops breathing for a few seconds and then makes this strangled sound and starts gasping like he's just run the marathon. I thought there was something seriously wrong with him at first.*
>
> Julia, 18 years

The first time

Most people never forget the first time they had intercourse, whether it was better than they expected, a disaster, or somewhere in between. It's impossible to get everything perfect the first time, but it helps if both partners are prepared and understand each other's needs.

THINKING AHEAD

The thought of having intercourse for the first time can be both exciting and frightening. Both of these emotions can make it difficult to relax, and can cause problems.

It is very important for anyone about to have sex to discuss contraception before they get carried away. Both girls and boys must take responsibility to avoid unwanted pregnancy and sexually transmitted disease. Alarmingly, statistics show that many couples don't use contraception or protection against infection the first time. However, there is *always* a risk of pregnancy and infection. Contraceptives are usually available free from a clinic and in some schools, and male condoms can be bought at a drugstore or supermarket.

Having to rush and worrying about privacy are common reasons for nervousness. For the first time, it helps to be somewhere comfortable and not in the back of a car. If your first experience is unplanned and unpleasant, forget it. Look forward to a "first time" having sex when conditions are right.

EXPECTATIONS AND REALITY

Most people want to "get it right," but what they think is right is likely to be based on films or books, and is probably not realistic. One of you might have had experience with another partner, or it may be the first time either person has seen another naked or touched anyone sexually. If the relationship is based on trust and respect and not just physical attraction, it can be wonderful. If it doesn't turn out as exciting as expected, don't worry – no one was ever an expert at anything at the first attempt.

THE IMPORTANCE OF AROUSAL

Men can be aroused just by thinking of sex or seeing their partner's body. A man may be so excited that he ejaculates before intercourse. A nervous man may find it difficult to get an erection. Kissing and caressing together should solve this.

Women generally take longer to become aroused to the point where the vagina opens up and produces lubricating

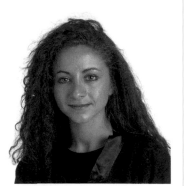

When we had sex the first time, I didn't enjoy the actual sex that much. What I did like was cuddling up to my boyfriend all night.

Josie, 17 years

IS IT EVER SAFE?

If you are not using any contraception, you can get pregnant even if:
- It is your first time.
- You made love standing up.
- Your monthly period has just finished.
- You wash out your vagina afterward.
- Your partner withdraws before ejaculation.
- You haven't had your first period.
- Your partner puts a condom on just before penetration (there may be some leakage of sperm beforehand).

fluid. The vagina may be closed or dry if a woman is nervous or not aroused. If the man is patient and asks what she likes, and if she can show or tell him, these problems can be avoided. If sex is painful, this is possibly because the vagina is not sufficiently lubricated. If extra lubrication is needed, special gels and lubricants are available at a drugstore. Be informed about what products are best: petroleum-based lubricants will destroy a male condom, for instance. Once a couple feel more confident, lubricant will not be needed.

BEING COMFORTABLE

Some girls feel pain the first time because their hymen is intact *(see page 15)*, and hurts when it is broken by intercourse. There may even be slight bleeding. It was once believed that a broken hymen meant a girl was not a virgin, but often the opening is either quite large or has been stretched in strenuous sports or by tampons. Others feel pain because they find it hard to relax the vaginal muscles – they need time to relax and feel comfortable.

The first time a couple has sex is often not spectacular; it takes time to get to know each other's bodies and to feel comfortable together. It should improve, but only if there is good communication and attention to each other's needs.

Men may thrust too deeply in the vagina; they should try to make sure that they are not hurting their partner. Most men will have an orgasm the first time they have intercourse, but most women will not. Like all things that need practice, sex usually gets better after the first time.

" I decided to wait until I was 18 before I had sex for the first time; I didn't feel ready before then. "
Peter, 18 years

" When I tried putting the condom on I just came right away. But we tried again later, and it was fine: I think I was calmer. "
Paul, 16 years

QUESTIONS AND ANSWERS

When you see sex in films, women always have orgasms, even the first time. When I had sex the first time, I was expecting fireworks, but nothing happened. Why not?
Terri, 16 years

Films are just unrealistic: most girls don't have an orgasm the first time that they have sex. It may take you time to learn how to respond to your boyfriend, and take him time to learn how to stimulate you to reach orgasm. Many girls and women do not have orgasms during intercourse at all unless they are very aroused, usually by having their clitoris stimulated at the same time. Sex improves with patience and practice.

I've just had sex with my girlfriend for the first time. I really wanted to look at her, but she said she felt too embarrassed. I don't get it – what's wrong with her?
Damon, 17 years

There is nothing wrong with her at all. Seeing your partner naked is very arousing for you, but some people are not used to being seen naked and feel embarrassed. She may be thinking of all the things she believes are wrong with her body. As time goes on, she will probably feel more relaxed and comfortable, and will start to enjoy you looking at, and being aroused by, her body – and looking at you.

Enjoying sex

Sexual enjoyment is all about giving and receiving pleasure, which means it is about communication. People reach orgasm in different ways, and to enjoy sex to the full, couples must tell one another what they like and – just as importantly – what they don't like.

REACHING ORGASM

Sometimes, a couple reach orgasm at the same time; more often, they don't. It doesn't really matter – whoever comes first can continue to stimulate the other to orgasm. Although orgasms are important to most people, they are not the only sexual sensation – there are plenty of others to enjoy.

VARIETY AND EXPERIMENTATION

Experimenting can be fun, provided that both partners are willing participants. Intercourse is not the only way of enjoying sex – foreplay, for example, can be continued until orgasm. This can be a choice for those who would rather postpone full penetrative sex. Other sexual activities can be as enjoyable as intercourse, and are safer, too, carrying little or no risk of pregnancy (*see page 70*) or of passing on infections (*see pages 80-83*).

TRYING DIFFERENT POSITIONS

Some couples always use the same position for sex; others vary their lovemaking. The many possible positions for intercourse can be divided into two primary groups: face to face and from

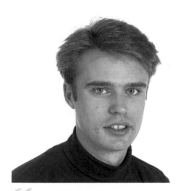

" We both decided to try out some different positions. Once I fell off the bed, but otherwise it's been a good experience. "

Charlie, 17 years

ANAL SEX

This is intercourse with the penis in the anus. Anal sex carries a high risk of infection including HIV if the sexual partner is infected (*see pages 84-85*), and a risk of other infections for women because the anus is full of bacteria that can be spread to the vagina by anal sex.

QUESTIONS AND ANSWERS

I have orgasms from masturbating or from oral sex, but never from intercourse. Will I ever be able to?
Tanya, 17 years

Many men and women think that if a man just thrusts away inside a woman long enough she will reach orgasm, but women rarely have orgasms during intercourse unless their clitoris is also stimulated. Some spend more time on foreplay, so that the woman becomes more aroused, and some women rub their clitoris themselves during intercourse. But don't see orgasm as the only goal; there are other enjoyable things about sex.

My boyfriend wants to tie me up when we have sex. I don't really want him to. What should I do?
Alex, 17 years

Sex is about doing what you *want* to do, and you should never be forced into doing anything that you don't want to. What your boyfriend wants to do is bondage, which some people – but not all – enjoy. Some enjoy the control of having sex with a person while they are in a submissive position. If you don't feel comfortable with this, and aren't prepared to be submissive, you don't have to do it: tell him firmly that you will not.

behind. In face-to-face positions, a couple can see, touch, and arouse one another. The most common position is with the man or woman on top; this is not necessarily the most satisfactory position for the woman because there is little clitoral stimulation. Other positions include side-by-side, seated, and standing. The chosen position is likely to be one that is comfortable for the individuals.

If the man enters the woman from behind, he can easily stimulate her breasts and clitoris. The most used position is often called the "doggie" position: the woman kneels on her hands and knees, and the man kneels behind her. Other positions include standing and side-by-side.

ORAL SEX

Oral sex means stimulating a partner's genitals with the lips and tongue. Couples may use oral sex as part of foreplay, or may continue to orgasm as an alternative to intercourse. Licking or kissing a woman's clitoris is called cunnilingus, while kissing and sucking a man's penis is known as fellatio. By being in control when stimulating the man, the woman can determine whether the man ejaculates in her mouth. Like all sexual contact, oral sex is more pleasant if the genitals are clean. Oral sex avoids the risks of pregnancy, but a genital infection or cold sores near the mouth can be transmitted during oral sex; there is also a risk of contracting HIV (*see page 84*).

> *Although I'm on the pill, I still get my boyfriend to wear a condom as well — for safer sex.*
>
> Cheryl, 17 years

POSITIONS FOR SEX

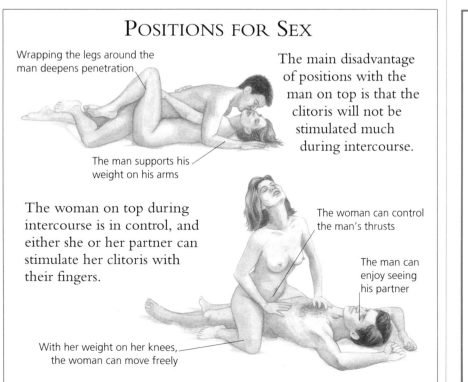

Wrapping the legs around the man deepens penetration

The main disadvantage of positions with the man on top is that the clitoris will not be stimulated much during intercourse.

The man supports his weight on his arms

The woman on top during intercourse is in control, and either she or her partner can stimulate her clitoris with their fingers.

The woman can control the man's thrusts

The man can enjoy seeing his partner

With her weight on her knees, the woman can move freely

GUIDELINES FOR EXPERIMENTATION

If you want to experiment with your sex life, you must be able to trust each other and you must be very clear about what you want.

■ Never be pushed into doing anything that you really don't want to do.
■ Never try to persuade an unwilling partner into doing anything: it isn't fair.
■ Agree in advance exactly what you want to do.
■ If your partner wants you to stop at any point, do so. You must respect their feelings and wishes.
■ Don't do anything that could be harmful or might hurt either of you.
■ Don't do anything that makes you feel ashamed — it isn't right for you.

Dealing with difficulties

It is not unusual to have sexual difficulties, whatever your age or experience. Sex is a sharing experience, not a test of your abilities, and a couple who have a good relationship can overcome most problems by talking them over.

WHY PEOPLE HAVE PROBLEMS

Any problems you might have will probably be caused by poor communication or inexperience, and most vanish with experience and better communication. Perhaps you are not yet ready for a sexual relationship and for the emotional issues of loyalty and commitment it involves. Some difficulties can be the result of anxiety – especially about being a "good performer" – and disappear once a person can relax. Other problems may result from guilt feelings or past experiences. If you think this is likely, it might be best to see a counselor.

PREMATURE EJACULATION AND ERECTION PROBLEMS

Premature ejaculation means coming too early, even before the penis is in the vagina. If the problem persists, the man can learn control by masturbating and stopping just before orgasm. Failure to get or maintain an erection happens to most men at some time, usually because they are tired or anxious or have drunk too much alcohol. Extra stimulation can help, but it may be better to try again later. Worrying about erection problems only makes them worse. If the problems do persist, talk to a doctor in case there is a medical reason.

NOT HAVING AN ORGASM

This is only a problem if it happens persistently. Not all women have orgasms every time they have sex. It takes time for them and their partners to learn how their bodies respond. Tension and anxiety can cause problems, too. Young men seldom have orgasm problems, although some older men do.

PAINFUL INTERCOURSE

If sex is painful for a woman, she may need more stimulation. Very rarely women may suffer from vaginismus, where the vaginal muscles tighten, making intercourse impossible. The woman should see her doctor if this persists. In uncircumcised men, a tight foreskin may make erection and intercourse painful, but this is rare *(see page 24)*. In both sexes, infections *(see pages 80-83)* can irritate the genitals so that intercourse is painful.

We'd had a great night and we were in bed but there was nothing happening – I'd had too much to drink. I was so embarrassed – she said I'd better cut down on beer in the future, or else!

Greg, 18 years

PREMATURE EJACULATION

This means coming before you want to and it is very common. It is often a shock and a disappointment to a man and his partner. It may happen the first few times you have sex, simply because you are experiencing the reality of sexual contact with another person. As you become used to being sexually excited by the sight and touch of your partner, you will gradually develop control of your ejaculation so that you can come when you want to. If you continue to come too quickly, don't feel a failure. If your partner is sympathetic, talk to her. Try different ways to make love that don't necessarily focus on you coming in her vagina.

CONTRACEPTION

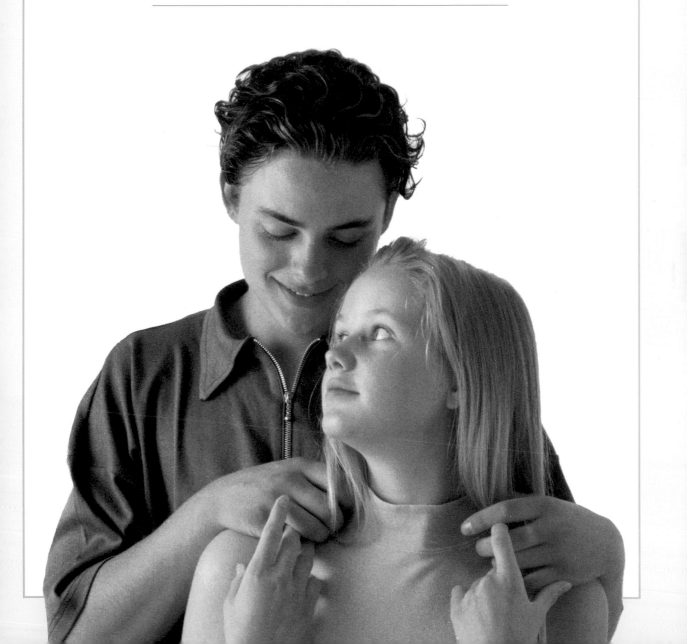

Choosing contraceptives

Contraceptives are used to prevent unplanned pregnancy. They are easy to get, free in many cases, and advice is confidential. From the very first sexual experience, both a man and a woman need to take responsibility for contraception.

RISK OF PREGNANCY

About half of all couples don't use contraceptives the first time they have sex. Some continue not using them, perhaps because they don't know where to get advice or feel too embarrassed to ask. They may think that contraception is the other person's responsibility. Many probably believe that they can get away with it, and some may want a child (*see page 70*). Those who have intercourse without contraception are always taking a risk. Without contraception, the probability of pregnancy is high, because fertility is highest in early adulthood.

WHERE TO GET CONTRACEPTIVES

Everyone is entitled to free, confidential advice on contraception from doctors (*see right*), family planning clinics. and in most schools. Condoms can be bought in supermarkets as well as drugstores and clinics. It may seem that it is premeditated and unspontaneous behavior to think about contraception before becoming sexually active, and many parents may even feel that this will lead to experimentation – but it isn't necessarily so. You and you alone are responsible for your body and what happens to it. Knowing about contraception is part of being responsible and taking control of your life.

Those who do plan in advance can discuss what type of contraceptive to use, and who is going to get it. Some couples visit a clinic or doctor together for advice and guidance. Advice is always confidential, so one can freely ask questions without any worries. Private doctors and doctors at clinics can prescribe most contraceptives. Some prefer not to go to a doctor, and buy condoms on their own.

TAKING THE LEAD
There is nothing to stop anyone from consulting a doctor or clinic about family planning, where condoms are usually free. It is completely unfair for boys to leave the contraception up to girls because they are the ones who get pregnant. Boys as well as girls who are going to be sexually active should ask themselves, "Am I ready to become a parent?"

The doctor will ask or may try to persuade those under 16 to tell their parents that they are using contraceptives; they are not legally required to inform them, but there is a chance they will. It is always best to discuss contraception with one's parents if at all possible — they may be glad to know that you are acting responsibly.

WHAT TO ASK FOR

The contraceptives that are supplied only by a doctor or clinic include the pill, cervical cap, diaphragm, intrauterine device, injectables, and implants. A doctor or clinic can also give advice about family planning. Family planning clinics will offer advice on the best method, based on a person's individual needs. Some methods are not suitable for young couples; some methods may affect one's health or may not be appropriate given a person's family medical history or habits, such as smoking. Those who are forgetful, for example, might not do well on a birth control pill that has to be taken at the same time every day.

Some routine tests may be made, such as a blood pressure check, and those who smoke may be advised to give it up. More than likely a pap smear will be taken, and followup visits will be scheduled to check that there are no side effects or problems connected to the contraception being used. Checkups every six months afterwards are advisable.

THE LAW AND CONTRACEPTION

Local laws may govern the age at which an adolescent can expect a medical consultation to be confidential. In some cases, a 16-year-old has a legal right to insist upon confidentiality. Contraception advice and contraceptives are available free from many schools and clinics for those who are reluctant to see a family doctor. Parental permission is not required to purchase any form of contraception.

QUESTIONS AND ANSWERS

I'm a virgin, but I want to start having sex. Can I use a diaphragm?
Janine, 16 years

If you use tampons, you may be able to use a diaphragm. Putting in a diaphragm takes practice, and if you feel nervous about sex at first, you may not want to have to worry about putting it in properly. You will be given a practice cap until you are confident.

Can you go on using the diaphragm when you have your period?
Paulette, 17 years

Yes. In fact, the diaphragm will contain bleeding temporarily while a couple make love. It must be left in place as usual after intercourse for at least six hours because there is a small chance that a girl can get pregnant during her period.

If I squirt spermicide into my vagina just before sex, will that kill the sperm?
Marsha, 16 years

No. Spermicides are sperm-killing chemicals but they are not effective enough on their own. They are used with barrier methods (*see pages 63-65*) as an extra precaution.

Why should there be female condoms if there are already male condoms? Is this a way to put the responsibility onto the woman?
Penny, 17 years

Taking responsibility for contraception is something that, ideally, everyone should do. This is a fairly new method of contraception and, like most methods, it takes time to get used to. Female condoms do protect against infection and unplanned pregnancy.

My boyfriend didn't want to use condoms, because he said they spoiled sex for him. I said no condom, no sex — the risk would spoil it for me.

Paula, 17 years

Types of contraceptives

Contraception has been used for over 3,000 years to prevent unplanned pregnancy. All forms of contraception work by preventing the fertilization of a woman's egg by a man's sperm. This is achieved in various ways.

Methods of contraception can be divided roughly into five groups. Barrier methods physically prevent sperm from swimming into the uterus and fertilizing the woman's egg (*see pages 60-65*); hormonal methods alter a woman's hormonal cycle to prevent fertilization (*see pages 58-59*); the intrauterine device (IUD) prevents the sperm from reaching the egg or may prevent the egg from embedding itself in the uterus (*see page 66*); natural methods are based on calculating the time when a woman is least fertile and abstaining or using another method to avoid conception when she is most fertile (*see page 67*); and sterilization is a permanent surgical means of preventing conception (*see page 67*). On the following pages, the advantages, disadvantages, and reliability of each of the contraceptive methods is given.

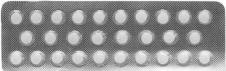

Progestogen-only pill

HORMONAL CONTRACEPTIVES
These work by introducing synthetic versions of female hormones into a woman's body. The hormones either stop her from ovulating, or make her cervical mucus thick, preventing sperm from reaching the uterus.
The hormones are taken by mouth, as an implant under the skin, or by injection.

Injectable hormone

Hormonal implants

INJECTIONS AND IMPLANTS
Some hormonal methods of contraception can only be administered by a doctor or a specially trained family planning nurse. These are injectable contraceptives and implants that have to be inserted under the skin. Both types are long-term and require no attention from the user.

Ring at open end

Female condom

Polyurethane sheath

Ring at closed end

MALE AND FEMALE CONDOMS
Condoms stop sperm from reaching the uterus. The male condom, made of thin rubber, is unrolled over the erect penis. The female condom, made of thin polyurethane, is inserted into the vagina. Whichever type is used by the couple must be put on, or inserted, before intercourse. Both types are thrown away after intercourse and can be used only once.

Flexible ring

Lubricated sheath

Male condom

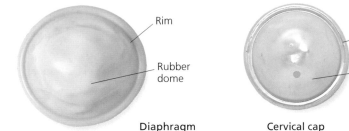

Rim

Rubber dome

Diaphragm

Rim

Rubber dome

Cervical cap

DIAPHRAGMS AND CERVICAL CAPS

These are inserted into the vagina before sex, where they cover the cervix and prevent sperm from reaching the uterus. The diaphragm and cervical cap, made of thin rubber, are used with a spermicide (*see below*), which increases the effectiveness of the method by killing any stray sperm. Both are left in place for several hours and are reusable after cleaning.

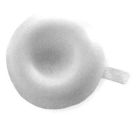

Spermicidal sponge

MORNING-AFTER PILL

Contraceptives can sometimes fail. If this happens, one should see a doctor or go to a clinic as soon as possible. The morning-after pill must be taken within 72 hours of unprotected intercourse to be effective. This emergency method must not be relied on as a regular contraceptive, however. It has only recently become available in the United States.

Vaginal suppositories containing spermicide

Spermicidal film

SPERMICIDES

These create a chemical barrier that kills or disables sperm in the vagina, so that the sperm don't reach the uterus. They are not an effective contraceptive on their own, however: they must always be used with another contraceptive, such as a cervical cap or diaphragm, to be effective. The spermicide is put into the vagina before intercourse. There are six main types: the spermicidal sponge, which is inserted into the vagina rather like a cap; vaginal suppositories and film, which melt inside the vagina; foam, which is squirted into the vagina; and creams and gels, which are used on diaphragms or cervical caps, or are squeezed into the vagina with a special applicator.

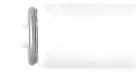

Spermicidal foam

Spermicidal cream

OTHER METHODS

There are other methods of contraception that are not recommended for young people. The intrauterine device, or IUD (*see page 66*), is a small piece of plastic with copper wire wrapped around it. It is inserted inside the uterus by a doctor, and prevents sperm from reaching the egg or a fertilized egg from settling. The IUD is not usually a first choice for young women who have not had children, because of the risk of infection. Sterilization operations (*see page 67*) permanently prevent women from becoming pregnant, or men from releasing sperm. Natural methods of contraception (*see page 67*) rely on knowing when the woman is fertile each month, and are extremely unreliable and difficult to practice.

IUD

Applicator used with spermicide

Hormonal methods

Because these contraceptives contain synthetic drugs that alter a woman's hormonal cycle, they are available only by prescription. Those who choose to use any of the hormonal methods will be asked to see a doctor regularly to have a general checkup.

WHAT IS THE BIRTH CONTROL PILL?

There are two basic types of pills. The combined pill contains low doses of the hormones estrogen and progestogen. This prevents ovulation (*see page 16*) so conception cannot take place. The progestogen-only pill contains progestogen. This pill causes the cervix to produce thick mucus, preventing sperm from entering the uterus; it may also prevent ovulation.

THE COMBINED PILL

The combined pill is taken each day for 21 days, followed by a seven-day break before starting the next pack. During the break some bleeding occurs. Women who like to take pills without a break can use a 28-pill pack that includes 21 pills with hormones, and seven pills without hormones. Bleeding occurs while these inactive "dummy" pills are taken.

ADVANTAGES AND DISADVANTAGES

The combined pill can be taken by most women, and it usually makes periods lighter and less painful. Because it is so reliable, the pill largely removes the fear of becoming pregnant, and helps many women and their partners feel more relaxed about sex. Before prescribing a contraceptive pill, a doctor will ask about a woman's health and that of her immediate family. This is because the pill may not be suitable for a woman if she, or members of her family, suffer from certain health problems, such as high blood pressure. It is also not suitable for smokers over 35, or very overweight women. Some women suffer side effects, such as headaches, or weight gain. If these do not go away, the woman should consult her doctor. Certain medication and a severe stomach upset – vomiting or severe diarrhea – can prevent the pill from working, and should be treated as a missed pill (*see opposite*).

THE PROGESTOGEN-ONLY PILL

The progestogen-only pill must be taken at the same time every day, without a break between packs. It is therefore not suitable for those who tend to be forgetful.

RELIABILITY

Hormonal methods are 99 percent effective if they are used carefully. Birth control pills are the best known of the hormonal methods and come in two basic forms. Effectiveness of the combined pill is reduced if pills are not taken as prescribed. Used carefully, the progestogen-only pill is only slightly less reliable than the combined pill. Injectable contraceptives are nearly 100 percent effective for the stated length of time – Depo-Provera up to 12 weeks and Noristerat up to 8 weeks.
Implants are nearly 100 percent effective.

ADVANTAGES AND DISADVANTAGES

The progestogen-only pill may cause periods to be irregular or missed – this is normal, but it should be mentioned to the doctor at a checkup. It is also suitable for women who cannot take estrogen. If taken more than three hours late, however, its effectiveness may be lost, and any vomiting or severe diarrhea will also stop it from working. Other methods of contraception would need to be used in this case.

THE INJECTABLE CONTRACEPTIVE

Progestogen is injected into the buttock and is released into the body over the following weeks. It works by preventing the release of an egg from the ovary each month. Injections are needed every eight or 12 weeks. There are two types of injection – Depo-Provera, which lasts for up to 12 weeks, and Noristerat, which lasts up to eight weeks.

Injectable contraception allows sex to be spontaneous and relieves the pressure of worrying about taking pills. The disadvantages are that possible side effects such as weight gain or irregular bleeding may occur until the drug wears off. Bleeding can be heavy at first, but most women have no bleeding after the second injection.

HORMONAL IMPLANTS

This is a fairly new method of hormonal contraception. Implants are plastic tubes, each tube about 1¼ in (34 mm) long and thinner than a matchstick, containing progestogen. Six tubes are inserted under the skin of a woman's upper arm. This is done under local anesthetic by a doctor, and takes about 10 minutes. The implant releases a constant supply of progestogen straight into the bloodstream for five years. Its effect can be reversed at any time by removing the tubes. Any side effects are the same as those for the progestogen-only pill.

MEMORY AID

To help you to remember to take your pill every day you should adopt a set routine. Always take it on waking or on going to bed at night. Follow the instructions and carry your pills with you in case you stay away for a night.

I told my girlfriend I didn't like her being on the pill, because it means that she could sleep with anyone. She told me I was being stupid.

David, 18 years

IF YOU FORGET A PILL

It is important that pills are taken on time and as prescribed. Pill packets come with instructions – read them carefully before starting on them and read them again to see what to do if a pill is late or missed. If in doubt, call your clinic or doctor. In the meantime, do not have sex. Also, do not "borrow" a birth control pill from someone else. Use only your own prescription.

QUESTIONS AND ANSWERS

Because I have painful periods, my doctor is going to put me on the pill. Is this a good idea?
Tracey, 14 years

Your doctor wouldn't prescribe the pill if you are likely to suffer any harmful side effects. Although you are on the contraceptive pill, this doesn't mean that you have to become sexually active right away. The pill is being prescribed to relieve your symptoms.

I am on the pill but I don't have one steady sexual partner, so I want to use a condom to prevent any infection. What should I say to my partner?
Janine, 18 years

It is a good idea to insist on using a condom while you are still experimenting with relationships. Tell your partner that using a condom protects you and him from sexually transmitted diseases.

Condoms

Both male and female condoms are easy to obtain and reliable if used properly. They can help to prevent not only pregnancy, but also the spread of sexually transmitted infections, including HIV. They also reduce the risk of cervical cancer in women *(see page 79)*.

THE MALE CONDOM

The male condom is usually made of very thin latex rubber, and fits snugly over the erect penis. When a man comes, or ejaculates, his semen stays inside the condom. Some condoms are made from animal tissues and are sold as a luxury item because they are supposed to "feel more natural." They are not effective enough to protect against pregnancy or infection. Condoms are also known by other names, including sheaths, rubbers, French letters, and johnnies.

Male condoms can be bought in drugstores and supermarkets, and can be obtained from family planning clinics, doctors, and in some schools. They come in different shapes and colors, with or without a tip at the end, and even in different flavors. Many are lubricated with spermicide to make them easier and safer to use. Check all condoms to make sure their expiration date has not passed and that they conform to current national or international safety standards.

THE FEMALE CONDOM

The female condom is a fairly new barrier method that can be bought in drugstores or obtained from some family planning clinics. It is a plastic tube that is bought ready lubricated; it fits inside the vagina, where it forms a lining into which the man directs his penis. One end is closed, and contains a ring to help keep it in place. The other end is held open with a similar ring that lies outside the vagina.

During sexual intercourse, when the woman's partner ejaculates inside her vagina, his semen is trapped inside the condom so that the sperm are prevented from swimming through the cervix and into her uterus.

BUYING AND USING CONDOMS

Some may be embarrassed about buying condoms at first, but stores sell them every day to people of all ages, and they can sometimes be found in dispensers in men's and even ladies' bathrooms. There are many different brands and types, so it helps to keep informed – a clinic can provide free information.

RELIABILITY

Female condoms are a relatively new method of contraception. They are thought to be as reliable as male condoms. Male condoms are between 85 and 98 percent effective, depending on care taken in handling them.

USING LUBRICANTS

Some couples prefer to use extra lubrication with condoms. Only spermicide creams or special gels should be used with male condoms. Products containing oil, such as baby oil, body lotions, and Vaseline, must *not* be used, because they can damage the rubber and make the condom leak. Female condoms are made of plastic, so any lubricants can be used with them.

USING A MALE CONDOM

The male condom is a convenient method of contraception. Putting on a condom need not be embarrassing and awkward. It can be part of the fun of foreplay if couples do it together.

Do not remove the condom until the penis has withdrawn from the vagina. Check it for any leakage and discard carefully after use – if possible, not in the toilet. Do not reuse.

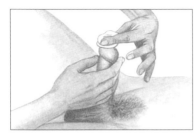

1 Whether you have a condom with or without a tip, squeeze the end to push out the air, so that there is space left for the sperm.

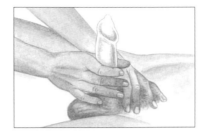

2 When the penis is erect, unroll the condom over the penis to the base. Doing this together can be fun.

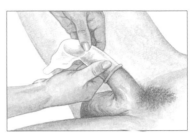

3 After ejaculation, the man holds the condom on his penis. Once he withdraws from the vagina, it can be taken off and discarded carefully.

USING A FEMALE CONDOM

The female condom is a fairly recent contraceptive. It is strong and comes ready lubricated. It also allows the woman to take the responsibility for safer sex. After use, check for any leakage and discard carefully.

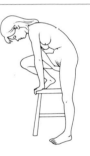

To insert the female condom, find a comfortable position to relax the vagina

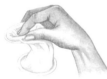

Squeeze the ring at the closed end into a narrow oval

1 Remove the condom from the packaging – it is already lubricated – and, with one hand, spread the labia (*see page 14*). With the other hand, slide the squeezed ring of the condom into your vagina, pushing it as far as possible.

2 With a finger inside the condom, maneuver the ring up past the pubic bone. The ring doesn't have to cover the cervix like a diaphragm does (*see page 64*). When in place, it should hang down about 2 in (5 cm) outside the vagina.

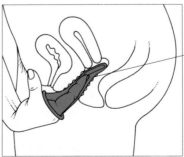

Push the closed end up into the vagina

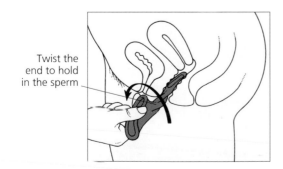

Twist the end to hold in the sperm

3 After sex, when the man's penis has been withdrawn, twist the open end of the condom to seal in the sperm. Pull the whole condom out of the vagina. Check the sheath for any leakages before discarding it. Do not use it again.

With practice, condoms are easy to use properly – try them out on your own first. Girls can practice putting a male condom on a banana or carrot.

Female condoms can be put in place anytime before sexual intercourse. Male condoms can only be put on when the penis is hard, and condoms must always be put on before any genital contact, because semen can leak from the penis before ejaculation. Two male condoms should *never* be used together for "extra" protection: they are likely to rub against each other and tear from friction.

After use, wrap the condom in tissue and throw it away carefully (not in the toilet). There will still be sperm on the penis, so it should be washed immediately and not brought near to the vagina until it has been washed. Condoms can only be used once; they must never be washed and used again because they will no longer protect against pregnancy or disease.

Advantages and disadvantages

Condoms are an effective way to practice safer sex. They reduce the risk of passing on or picking up a number of sexually transmitted infections and diseases (*see pages 80-83*), including the virus that causes AIDS. Condoms should be treated carefully, though: jagged nails, rings, or teeth used to rip open the packet can tear them.

A male condom might split or slip off, especially if the man doesn't hold the condom as he pulls his penis out of his partner's vagina. When using the female condom, the penis could slip outside the condom so that ejaculation takes place in the vagina. In either situation, as soon as possible see a doctor, who may prescribe the morning–after pill (*see page 66*).

QUESTIONS AND ANSWERS

I carry a condom around with me but my friends think that I'm playing easy to get. How can I argue that I am right and that I'm not looking for sex all the time?
Miriam, 17 years

This double standard in which women are regarded differently from men has always existed (*see page 36*). HIV and AIDS have changed views about carrying and using condoms. By carrying one "in case," you are acting sensibly and realistically. You are showing that you care about your sexual health and that of your partner. It's better to be safe than sorry!

If I use a condom, when is the best time to put it on?
Pete, 16 years

The best time to do this is early on while you still have a cool enough head to get everything right. This is another argument for doing it together – having fun and being responsible, rather than rushing. The male condom must be put on when your penis is erect. If you wait too long, you may be too physically close to your partner to stop and open a packet and put the condom on. Putting it on too late may cause you to come early.

Barrier methods

A diaphragm is used with spermicide and is put into the vagina before sex. When the man ejaculates, his sperm cannot swim into the woman's uterus, because the diaphragm blocks its entrance, and the sperm are killed by the chemicals in the spermicide.

DIAPHRAGM AND CERVICAL CAP

Both these contraceptives are made of thin rubber, and both cover the cervix. The more popular of the two is the diaphragm; it is a dome, 2-4 in (5-10 cm) across, with a springy rim. The cervical cap is smaller and fits over the cervix in the same way that a thimble fits over a finger. Diaphragms and cervical caps come in various sizes, and a doctor or nurse has to make sure that the size is right and demonstrate how to use it. Diaphragms and cervical caps are available from doctors or family planning clinics; they are also available from drugstores, but then the size needs to be known.

The diaphragm or cervical cap is removed by hooking a finger over the rim. It can be cleaned in warm water and mild soap, dried, and used again. It should be checked regularly for holes by holding it up to a bright light. The fit needs to be checked by a doctor or nurse about every 12 months. Gaining or losing more than 7 lb (3 kg) in weight, or having a baby, an abortion or a miscarriage, may change the shape of a woman's vagina, making a new diaphragm or cervical cap necessary.

HOW TO USE A DIAPHRAGM OR CERVICAL CAP

Both a diaphragm and a cervical cap must *always* be used with spermicides. With a diaphragm, the spermicide is smeared all over; with a cervical cap, it is smeared on both sides, but not around the rim. A diaphragm or cervical cap can be inserted at any time before intercourse – if it is more than three hours before, some extra spermicide should be inserted in the vagina before intercourse. After intercourse, the diaphragm or cervical cap should be left in place for at least six hours, or sperm left in the vagina may swim into the uterus. For repeated intercourse, more spermicide is needed in the vagina each time, although the diaphragm or cervical cap need not be removed.

ADVANTAGES AND DISADVANTAGES

The diaphragm or cervical cap is used only during sex, and it also helps to protect women against cervical cancer and some sexually transmitted infections. There are no side effects and

---

RELIABILITY

Used carefully, diaphragms and cervical caps are 98 percent effective, but their reliability can drop to 85 percent with less careful use. Spermicide alone is not recommended as an effective contraceptive.

" My friend wanted to borrow my diaphragm. I told her no, because diaphragms are like clothes – you need a size that fits you. Anyway, who wants to share something that goes inside you? "

Lorraine, 16 years

INSERTING A DIAPHRAGM

The diaphragm is made of rubber. It is placed in the vagina so that it covers the cervix. This means that no sperm can travel into the uterus. Spermicide, which contains chemicals that kill the sperm, is always used as an extra precaution with a diaphragm.

Find a comfortable position to relax the vagina

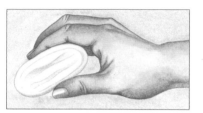

1 Wash hands and remove the diaphragm from its container. Squeeze the flexible rim into an oval shape with the index finger on top to keep the springy rim under control.

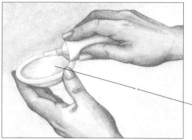

Smear two 1 in (3 cm) strips of spermicide on both sides of the diaphragm

2 Smear the spermicide in two strips (about 1 in/3 cm long) onto both sides of the diaphragm and around the rim. It will be slippery and quite difficult to handle.

Insert the diaphragm into the vagina

3 Insert the flexible rim of the diaphragm as high as it will go into the vagina. The direction is the same as that when a tampon is inserted – upward and backward.

Check that the diaphragm covers the cervix

4 Once the diaphragm is in place, it is held over the cervix by its springy rim. Check this by feeling for the cervix through the rubber with a finger. The cervix feels like the end of the nose.

TOXIC SHOCK

A few years ago some women who were using a highly absorbent tampon (no longer available) suffered a dangerous condition called toxic shock syndrome. The tampons were changed less often, and this encouraged growth of a bacterium in the vagina. There are no real risks in using ordinary tampons, a cervical cap or diaphragm, but six hours is the maximum time for leaving a tampon in the vagina (see pages 16-17).

INSERTING A CERVICAL CAP

The cap is thimble-shaped and smaller than the diaphragm. It stays in place over the cervix by suction. Spermicide should be put inside the cervical cap but not around the rim because this might affect the suction. Like all methods, this requires practice to get it right. Often you will be given a practice cervical cap to help you to feel confident about inserting it.

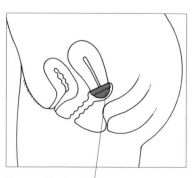

The cap fits directly over the cervix

no health risk from using the diaphragm or cervical cap, although with their use, cystitis (*see page 82*) is more common and there may be an occasional allergic reaction to the rubber. The woman must plan ahead and carry her diaphragm or cervical cap with her. Putting this contraceptive in place takes experience to ensure it is inserted properly. Many people find the spermicide messy and distracting.

Although the cervical cap or diaphragm must be left in the vagina for up to six hours after sexual intercourse, it should not be left there for any longer. Anything that is left in the vagina for too long – for 24 hours or more – which includes a tampon, may lead to a dangerous condition called toxic shock syndrome (*see opposite*).

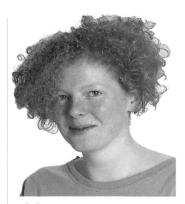

The first time I tried to put my diaphragm in, it slipped out of my fingers, flew across the room, and bounced off the wall. We just couldn't stop laughing, and it really helped us relax.

Polly, 17 years

USING SPERMICIDES

Most spermicides contain the chemical nonoxynol, which kills not only sperm, but also the organisms that cause many sexually transmitted infections, including HIV. They are not very effective as a contraceptive on their own, however. After intercourse, it is better not to have a bath for about six hours, because this may dilute spermicide or wash it away. A shower is a better option. Spermicide comes in different forms, including the sponge (*see below*); vaginal suppositories, which melt in the vagina; gels or creams, which are smeared over the diaphragm; foam, which is squirted into the vagina from an aerosol; and film, which dissolves in the vagina. All can be bought at drugstores or obtained from a doctor or family planning clinic.

THE SPONGE

The sponge is soft and round, about 2 in (5 cm) wide, and is made of foam soaked with spermicide. It has a dimple on one side, which fits over the cervix, and a loop attached to the other side, used to remove it. Before use, the sponge is first moistened with water in order to release the spermicide. It is then pushed, dimple side up, to the top of the vagina. The dimple should fit over the cervix. The sponge works for up to 24 hours, and it should be left in place for six hours after the last sexual intercourse. It is removed by pulling on the loop. It is not reusable.

WHICH SPERMICIDE?

The sponge is available over the counter, and its spermicide action remains effective no matter how many times intercourse occurs in a 24-hour period. It can be quite expensive, however, since a sponge only lasts one day. Many women prefer to use a form of spermicide that fits easily into a bag or purse.

Other methods

There are other contraceptive options available, but not generally recommended for the young. These include intrauterine devices, permanent sterilization, and natural methods. The morning-after pill can be used in an emergency, not as a regular method.

THE INTRAUTERINE DEVICE (IUD)

Most IUDs (previously known as the coil) are pieces of plastic, 1-1½ in (2-4 cm) long, wound with copper wire. The IUD works mainly by preventing sperm from reaching the egg, or rarely, by preventing a fertilized egg from settling in the uterus. The IUD is inserted into the uterus by a doctor using a special instrument. It can stay there for five years and is removed by a doctor.

An IUD is not chemical, it doesn't interfere with sexual intercourse, and it is effective as soon as it is fitted. However, IUDs may increase the risk of sexually transmitted infection in the uterus or the fallopian tubes – infection that could lead to infertility. This is one reason why they are generally not recommended for young women. Periods can be heavier, and it is possible for the IUD to become dislodged; it should be checked regularly by feeling for the tail of threads at the cervix. There have been some serious problems with IUDs in the past.

RELIABILITY

The IUD is more than 98 percent reliable. Sterilization for women is nearly 100 percent reliable once a woman has had her first period after the operation, and, for men, within a few months – the time it takes for the sperm to be cleared from the tubes. Natural methods are about 80 to 98 percent effective if used properly.

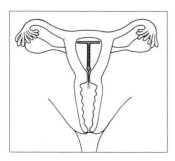

THE IUD IN PLACE
Two fine threads attached to the base of the IUD project a short way into the vagina. The woman can check, by putting a finger in her vagina and feeling for the threads, that the IUD is still in place.

EMERGENCY CONTRACEPTION

Emergency or post-coital (after intercourse) contraception, also known as the morning-after pill, is used when a woman thinks she is at risk of an unplanned pregnancy soon after intercourse. The reason could be forgetting to use contraception, an accident such as a condom tearing or slipping off, or that a woman was not planning to have sex – this includes sexual assault and rape. In such situations, one must contact a doctor or family planning clinic within 72 hours of the unprotected intercourse. The treatment generally consists of two special pills to take immediately, and another two to take 12 hours later. The pills alter a woman's hormonal balance, which delays ovulation or prevents implantation. They can also cause a sick feeling, or vomiting, which could mean that more pills must be taken. This method is about 95 to 99 percent effective. Another method in emergencies for older women is to have an IUD fitted, which can be done up to five days after unprotected intercourse. This prevents the egg from embedding itself in the uterine lining. The IUD can be removed when the next period starts. This is almost 100 percent effective in preventing pregnancy and is chosen if the time limit for the hormonal method has passed or the woman cannot take estrogen.

STERILIZATION

Male sterilization, or vasectomy, is done by cutting the sperm duct, or vas deferens *(see page 25);* this prevents sperm from reaching the penis. Female sterilization is done by cutting or blocking the fallopian tubes *(see page 15),* preventing eggs from reaching the uterus. Neither affects the person's interest in, or ability to enjoy, sex. A man still ejaculates semen (without the sperm) and a woman still has periods. These operations are designed to be irreversible. Doctors generally sterilize only men or women over 30 who have completed their family.

NATURAL METHODS

Often called the rhythm method, the natural method is extremely unreliable because it is so difficult to chart precisely a woman's fertile time, Natural methods depend on careful monitoring, finding out when a woman ovulates *(see pages 16-17).* During the fertile part of the cycle, other barrier forms of contraception or abstinence should be used. To be effective, the methods must be taught by a trained teacher and not tried without instruction.

TAKING TEMPERATURES

Temperature changes, measured with a fertility thermometer at the same time each day before getting out of bed (either orally, rectally, or vaginally), show when a woman is fertile. The fertility thermometer has a narrow range of temperatures, making it easy to read. Immediately after ovulation, the body temperature drops a little and then rises by between 0.2°F and 0.4°F. It remains at this temperature until the next period.

> ❝ *My friend had sex without using a contraceptive. She asked me if she could take some of my pills to stop her from getting pregnant. I said it wouldn't work, and she should see her doctor.* ❞
>
> Susan, 17 years

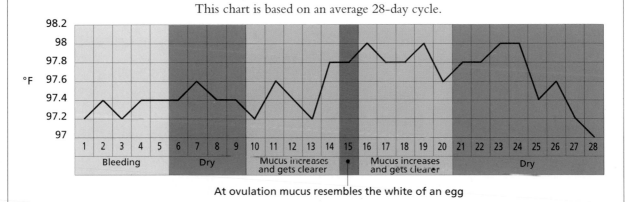

USING THE NATURAL METHOD

A daily record in chart form of temperature and/or cervical mucus must be kept for this method. Day 1 is the first day of bleeding.

Depending on the length of the cycle, ovulation should occur 12-16 days *before* the next period is due.

This chart is based on an average 28-day cycle.

°F

98.2 98 97.8 97.6 97.4 97.2 97

| 1 | 2 | 3 | 4 | 5 | 6 | 7 | 8 | 9 | 10 | 11 | 12 | 13 | 14 | 15 | 16 | 17 | 18 | 19 | 20 | 21 | 22 | 23 | 24 | 25 | 26 | 27 | 28 |

Bleeding   Dry   Mucus increases and gets clearer   Mucus increases and gets clearer   Dry

At ovulation mucus resembles the white of an egg

CERVICAL MUCUS METHOD

Changes in the consistency of a woman's cervical mucus *(see page 17)* also indicate ovulation. One can stretch a little vaginal discharge between the thumb and index finger to see the color and consistency. Immediately after a period, there may not be much cervical mucus. After a few days, the cervical mucus may be more noticeable as a discharge; it is thick, sticky, and cloudy. As one is about to ovulate and after ovulation, there is more mucus, and it is clear and stretchy – like raw egg white. When it changes back to being thick and cloudy, this is a "safe" time.

ADVANTAGES AND DISADVANTAGES

Natural family planning has been practiced for centuries, and it has no known side effects. Both the man and woman need to be involved and be prepared to use barrier methods or abstain at other times to be sure. It does require a detailed knowledge of a woman's cycle, and this record keeping is time-consuming and must be precise. Some say that those who practice the rhythm method or natural family planning need to be fully prepared to become parents.

"BEING CAREFUL" OR COITUS INTERRUPTUS

Coitus interruptus or withdrawal is when the man withdraws his penis from the vagina just before orgasm. This is not at all reliable as birth control because some sperm can leak before ejaculation; one sperm is all that is necessary for a pregnancy. Other disadvantages are that this is a difficult thing to do in practice, and the experience for both partners can be frustrating and unsatisfactory.

QUESTIONS AND ANSWERS

What if I were sterilized now and have it undone when I am older and want a family?
Kenny, 16 years

When you are young, a doctor would be very unlikely to consider sterilization unless your health were at risk. If you are sterilized, complicated surgery is required to reverse the sterilization operation. After sterilization, you are still exposing yourself and your partner to sexually transmitted infections and diseases *(see pages 80-83)* if you never use any other form of contraception, such as a condom.

I've heard that if you shake up a bottle of warm cola or any carbonated drink, and squirt it up into your vagina after you have sex, it will stop you from getting pregnant because it washes all the sperm back out. Is this true?
Lucy, 15 years

No, this will not prevent you from becoming pregnant. Washing out the vagina like this is called douching. By the time you start douching after you've had sex, the sperm will already be swimming into the uterus. Douching after sex can cause irritation or an infection in your vagina.

PREGNANCY AND BEING A PARENT

- How pregnancy starts
- Childbirth
- Unplanned pregnancy

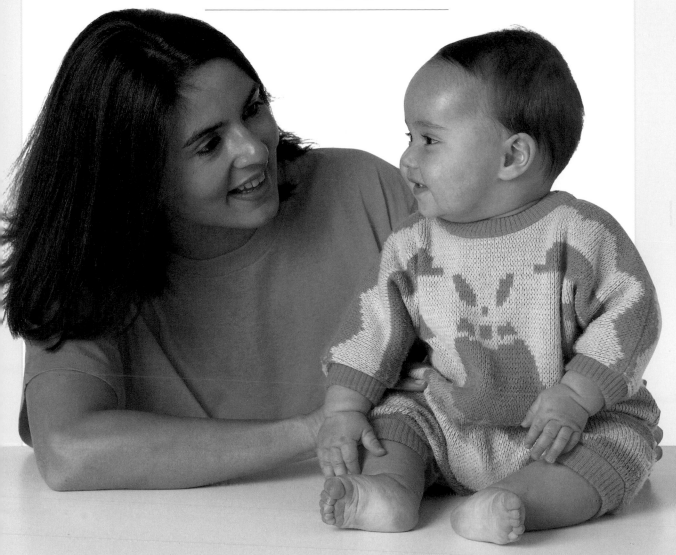

How pregnancy starts

The moment of fertilization, when egg and sperm fuse together, is the most significant event in the whole reproductive process. All the material is there for a new individual, who inherits genes from both parents.

About every 28 days – although it can actually be anywhere between 21 and 42 days – from puberty to menopause, an egg, or ovum, is released from a woman's ovaries *(see page 15)*. If she has intercourse around this time, there is a good chance that her partner's sperm will meet and fertilize the egg, beginning the process of conception. The process is complete when the ball of cells that develops from the fertilized egg attaches itself to the wall of the uterus. At first, this implanted mass of cells is called an embryo. Some of the cells develop into the placenta, which anchors the embryo in the uterus wall and delivers nutrition from the mother. A cushioning bag of fluid, called the amniotic sac, forms around the embryo. Eight weeks after fertilization, the embryo has a recognizable form, with face and limbs and all its major organs. It is now called a fetus. The baby will be born about 40 weeks after the first day of the woman's last period.

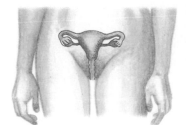

EXPANSION OF THE UTERUS
The uterus is about 4 in (10 cm) long, and 3 in (8 cm) wide. In pregnancy, its capacity and muscle bulk increase until it is about 15 in (38 cm) long and 10 in (25 cm) wide.

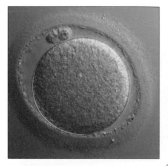

Hundreds of sperm surround the ripe egg, all trying to break through. The sperm release an enzyme, which dissolves the covering of the egg so that one sperm eventually penetrates it. Once this happens, no other sperm can get through. The fertilized egg, called a zygote, has 46 chromosomes – 23 from the sperm and 23 from the egg

BOY OR GIRL?

A baby's gender depends on the sperm. Genetic information, including sex, is carried in chromosomes – there is an identical set of 46 of these in every cell of the body, but eggs and sperm have only 23 each. Sperm can carry an X chromosome or a Y chromosome. The egg only carries an X chromosome. If a Y sperm fertilizes an egg, the baby's cells will be XY, and it will be a boy. If the sperm is X, the baby's cells will be XX, and it will be a girl.

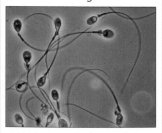

A sperm's head carries the genetic information, and its long tail propels it.

QUESTIONS AND ANSWERS

Can a girl get pregnant the first time she has sex?
Nathan, 13 years

Yes: whether it's the first time or the twenty-first, she can get pregnant if the couple doesn't use contraception.

If a girl misses a period, is she definitely pregnant?
Sarah, 14 years

No. Girls often have irregular periods, so being late, or even missing a period, is not uncommon. The only reliable way to find out is to have a pregnancy test *(see page 74)* if pregnancy is a possibility.

A pregnancy test is able to detect a certain hormone in a woman's urine. This is usually possible within a week of a missed period. However, whatever the result, it is advisable to visit a doctor or clinic to have the result confirmed.

A friend told me that you can't get pregnant if you have sex during your period – is she right?
Alison, 15 years

No. Ovulation can happen shortly after a period, and sperm can live to find an egg for up to three days, so a girl certainly can become pregnant if she has sex during her period.

One and a half days after fertilization, the fertilized egg has split into two connected cells, the first of a series of divisions that create the billions of cells in a baby's body. Each cell contains the full set of 46 chromosomes, which will be duplicated in all the cells that form. They carry genes, which determine or influence people's appearance and characteristics

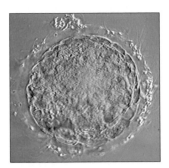

Three days after fertilization, more cell divisions have produced a solid mass of 64 separate cells. This ball of cells, which is called a morula, is no bigger than the period at the end of this sentence. It is still traveling down the fallopian tube and will not reach the uterus for another 24 hours

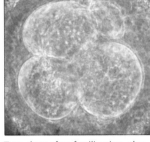

Two days after fertilization, the journey down to the uterus continues. A second split has taken place, producing four cells. From now on, the cells will divide about twice every day

Fallopian tube

Thickened by hormones, the uterine lining is ready to receive the egg

An egg has around 12-24 hours in which to be fertilized after ovulation

Ovary

THE STAGES OF CONCEPTION

During intercourse *(see pages 46-47)*, up to 500 million sperm are released from the penis. The sperm swim into the uterus and toward the ovaries – only a few thousand will make it this far. If they find an egg, they will surround it, and there is a good chance that one of them will fertilize it. The fertilized egg divides into a mass of cells as it travels down the fallopian tube. It attaches itself to the inside of the uterus, and at this site, the placenta begins to grow. The uterus keeps its lining, which is usually shed in menstruation, so the first sign of pregnancy is normally a missed period. Over the next 266 days, the tiny ball of cells develops at a rapid rate into a fully formed baby.

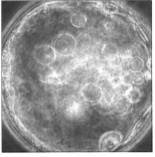

One week after fertilization a hollow space has formed in the center of the ball of cells, now called a blastocyst. After floating in the uterus for two or three days, it starts to embed itself in the wall. When the blastocyst is fully implanted, conception is complete

Childbirth

After about 40 weeks, a pregnancy comes to an end when the baby is born. The sequence of events that leads to the birth is called labor — divided into three stages — during which the uterus contracts with increasing strength and pushes the baby and placenta out.

Regular contractions of the uterus are a sign that labor has begun. It is time to contact the doctor and go to the hospital where arrangements have already been made for the birth. A nurse usually carries out routine examinations. The father or a close friend or relative is usually present throughout the labor. Labor is painful, as contractions of the uterus increase in frequency and intensity. The woman can feel tired, and frightened at this time, but breathing exercises help. During the birth, she may experience extreme pain, although procedures learned at prenatal classes or painkilling drugs will help lessen the pain and reduce fear. The support and encouragement of those with her is very important. During the second stage of labor the baby is born; the doctor assesses its health and hands the baby to the mother. Returning home can be a letdown. After all the congratulations comes the responsibility of taking care of the new arrival. Parents may feel exhausted from lack of sleep, and mothers can feel especially lonely during the first months. Support from a partner, family, and friends is important at this time. It can also be helpful and reassuring to meet other young parents to share ideas and problems.

DEVELOPMENT OF THE FETUS

At 16 weeks, the mother will notice changes to her breasts. The fetus has started to move. Its heartbeat can be heard. By 20 weeks, the mother begins to look pregnant, and she can feel the fetus moving inside her. At 32 weeks, the fetus is completely formed, and if born now, it has a 50 percent chance of survival. In the remaining 8 weeks it will put on fat, becoming plumper and less wrinkled.

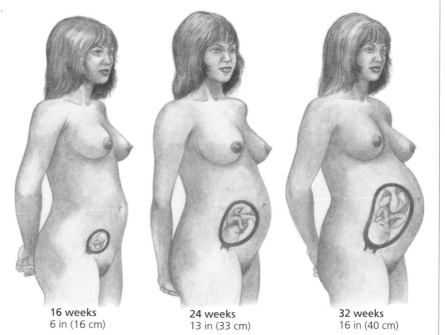

16 weeks
6 in (16 cm)

24 weeks
13 in (33 cm)

32 weeks
16 in (40 cm)

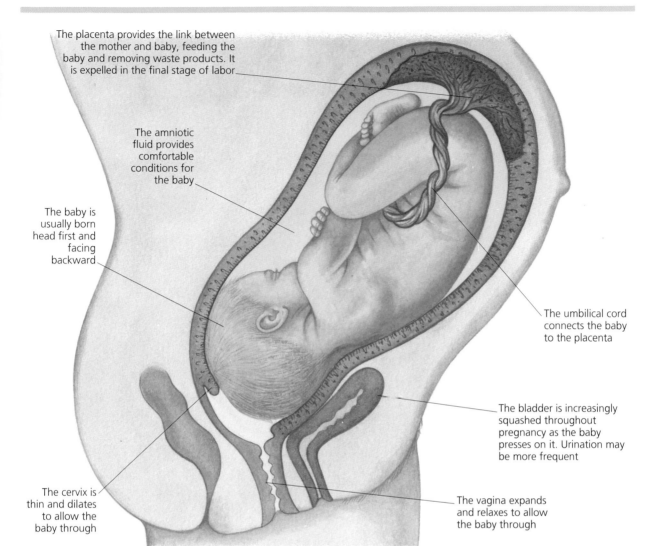

The placenta provides the link between the mother and baby, feeding the baby and removing waste products. It is expelled in the final stage of labor

The amniotic fluid provides comfortable conditions for the baby

The baby is usually born head first and facing backward

The umbilical cord connects the baby to the placenta

The bladder is increasingly squashed throughout pregnancy as the baby presses on it. Urination may be more frequent

The cervix is thin and dilates to allow the baby through

The vagina expands and relaxes to allow the baby through

THE PELVIC GIRDLE

During birth, the baby has to pass through a narrow opening in the pelvic girdle, a ring of bone consisting of the hip bones and lower spine, held together by tough ligaments. In fact, the baby is only able to squeeze through the narrow opening because hormones (also released throughout pregnancy) relax the ligaments, making the pelvic girdle wider and more flexible so that it "gives" as the baby is born.

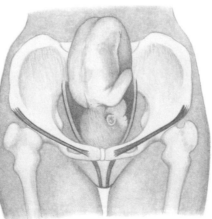

This is a front view of the baby's position in the pelvic girdle, with the uterus left out for clarity.

READY FOR THE BIRTH

Labor has three stages. The first stage generally lasts between 12 and 14 hours, although this time can vary. The uterus contracts strongly and frequently. The bag of fluid surrounding the baby bursts, and the cervix opens up (dilates) to allow the baby's head to pass through. The cervix should be fully dilated before the second stage begins. As the woman pushes downward and her uterus contracts more strongly, the baby is born. After delivery, the umbilical cord is clamped and cut. During the final stage, which lasts about 15 minutes, the placenta is pushed out of the uterus.

Unplanned pregnancy

It's easy to think that this can't happen, but it can be devastating to find out that it has. Once a young woman is pregnant, it may be hard to think of anything except how to tell one's parents, but there are many other decisions that also need to be made.

WHAT TO DO FIRST

To help you to sort out your feelings about the pregnancy, ask yourself the following questions first:
- Do you want the baby?
- Will your parents be supportive of your decision?
- Do you want your partner to be involved?
- Do you think your partner will stand by you?
- Is there someone you can confide in?
- Would you consider an abortion?
- Would you consider adoption?

FACING UP TO BEING PREGNANT

A girl discovering that she is pregnant may feel frightened, angry, and fearful about the future. The first step is to think through all the issues concerning the pregnancy, the baby, and what the future holds. It is very important to act quickly and to seek help and advice.

The choices facing a pregnant girl are not easy. She should not be pressured into doing what someone else thinks is right. Whatever choice she makes, it has to be right for her. Her partner may want to share in the decisions, but might not be ready for the responsibility, or be much help. He may be another complication in her life. He may not want to know. In the end, what happens must be the girl's choice. Her partner's agreement is not legally necessary for the continuation or termination of a pregnancy. Once a baby is born, if the father's name is on the birth certificate, he has legal rights and responsibilities that may include financial support of the mother and the baby.

TELLING THE MOTHER'S PARENTS

Every pregnant girl needs support and advice, especially in making the decision about telling her parents. Even in the closest families this can be difficult. Some find that talking first to a trusted family member or friend helps, and that they can suggest how to approach one's family. For a girl who can't tell her parents, the best place to turn to may be a family planning clinic, health center, or counseling service (*see pages 92-93*). The people there are trained to offer help and advice; they won't pass judgments or criticize. But in seeking advice, be careful to go to an organization that does not try to coerce a girl either into having the baby or seeking a termination.

BEING TOGETHER Once the baby is born, many girls find that they can cope as well as women twice their age, and enjoy motherhood.

CHOOSING TO HAVE THE BABY

A girl who is in a stable relationship, or who has family willing to help and support her, might keep the baby. This would mean rethinking one's whole future. Babies are not babies for long: a girl deciding to have a baby should try to imagine how she will feel bringing up a child for the next 16 or so years. Those who are very young, or on their own, may find this very difficult economically and emotionally. The opportunity for a girl to continue her schooling under these circumstances will depend to a large degree on her family and how they support her and the baby – whether financially, or by providing housing and childcare. The cooperation of the school system will also be important.

Having the baby and giving it up for adoption is another option. It is difficult for a girl to know how she will feel when the baby is actually born: some mothers find that they cannot give the baby up. Others decide to go through with it, although they often change their minds once the process is under way.

Once the pregnancy starts to show, some girls decide to leave school and make arrangements to continue with their education at home until the birth. Those who want to continue their studies after the baby is born may find that their family can help arrange childcare, or there may be a program in their school or neighborhood for young mothers and babies.

BEING A SINGLE PARENT

Bringing up a child alone is not easy. It can be harder still when all one's friends are still carefree teenagers. Money and housing are often problems. Family support can make a significant difference. Family members may be able to help out financially, but, just as importantly, they can provide emotional support and practical help. Even when parents are upset or angry about an unexpected pregnancy, they are still family, and it is worth trying to build bridges and maintain a good relationship with them.

HAVING THE PREGNANCY TERMINATED (ABORTION)

Abortion is the medical term for the termination of a pregnancy. Abortion raises many issues. It is legal in Canada and has been legal in the US since 1973. It is performed by a variety of methods. Most people have a view on whether it is an appropriate course of action or not. Remember, though, it is the girl's body involved, and it is her decision to make.

The earlier an abortion is performed, the safer it is. An abortion cannot be performed after 24 weeks except under exceptional circumstances. Vacuum aspiration, also called "D & C," is the most common method of abortion used until about 12 weeks. Under general anesthetic, the cervix is dilated

> ❝ *The worst part was telling Mom and Dad. Once I'd done that, it was easier to think clearly about what I wanted to do.* ❞
>
> Amy, 16 years

PREGNANCY TEST

A variety of pregnancy testing kits are available from drugstores. One type consists of a strip impregnated with chemicals. This is held in the woman's urine for a few seconds, and if it changes color, she is pregnant. These kits are 99 percent accurate, but results should be confirmed by a doctor or at a clinic. There are a number of agencies that offer free pregnancy testing services, and they can also provide free advice about contraception if you are not pregnant *(see pages 92-93)*.

and the uterine lining is sucked out through a small plastic tube. This takes about 10 minutes.

In more advanced pregnancies (12–20 weeks), abortion can be accomplished by the insertion of a prostaglandin suppository against the cervix. This hormone stimulates the pregnant uterus to contract much as it does in labor. Abortion often occurs within several hours, although repeat insertions may be necessary to complete the process. This can be upsetting because it is like a real birth, so the earlier the abortion is arranged, the better. In later pregnancies, the cervix is dilated under general anesthetic and an instrument is used to scrape out the fetal tissues.

Before a girl becomes pregnant, she may have strong views on whether or not she would ever have an abortion. But she could feel differently once she is actually pregnant, and so could her partner. A girl thinking of having an abortion should see her own doctor or a doctor at a family planning clinic as soon as possible so she can make an informed decision early in the pregnancy.

THE AFTERMATH

After an abortion a girl may feel relieved, or she may not feel as pleased as she thought she would. Even when a girl believed this way was the correct course of action, she may experience a great sense of loss. The best thing to do is to talk to someone sympathetic, such as a friend or a counselor at a family planning clinic. Don't hold feelings in – seek support at this difficult time. It is also important to seek advice on the type of contraception to use in the future (*see pages 56-57*).

ABORTION LAW

Abortion is legal in Canada, and in the US since 1973. Many states require a 24-hour waiting period between counseling sessions and the abortion, parental consent for girls under 18, and counseling by a doctor on alternatives to abortion. In some states, judicial approval can replace parental consent when the young woman involved cannot or will not obtain parental consent. Parental consent is required for a minor's abortion in 23 states. Other states have similar laws that are not being enforced because of court injunctions.

QUESTIONS AND ANSWERS

My boyfriend's always been a bit wild. I would really like to have a baby with him. Do you think it would settle him down?
Angela, 17 years

It's just as likely to make him leave. Have a baby when your relationship works, not to make it work.

I am pregnant, and I don't want to tell the baby's father because it is all over between us. My parents think I should. Is telling him the right thing to do?
Lee, 18 years

This is a difficult decision if your relationship is over but you have decided to keep the baby. If possible, your ex-boyfriend should really be told about the baby as he is the father. What you decide to do, however, is still up to you and not to him.

I think I'm pregnant. I still live at home: if I go to a clinic for a test, will they tell my parents?
Tina, 16 years

No: if you are pregnant, it will be up to you to tell your parents. In the case of abortion, however, some states require parental consent.

Sex and Health

Taking care of your body

Diseases and infections

HIV and AIDS

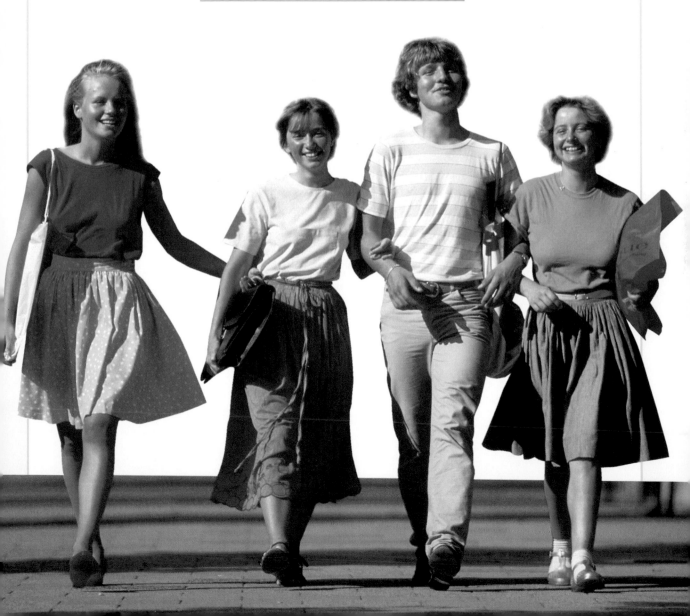

Taking care of your body

In adolescence, your body changes in ways that affect not just your appearance, but your health and personal hygiene too. Your skin produces new smells, your genitals secrete new substances, and you have to start taking care of your body in a different way.

PERSONAL SCENT

Everyone has their own smell. If you are clean and healthy, it's natural and pleasant, and a part of you. Animals secrete scent chemicals called pheromones, which help to attract mates. It is possible that we secrete pheromones, too, and that when we are attracted to someone, we may be responding to them by secreting these substances.

When body secretions have been exposed to air for a while, they become breeding grounds for bacteria and have an unpleasant smell. Almost everyone uses deodorants and antiperspirants (*see page 10*) to counteract underarm odors. Daily washing of the genital area is also essential. A different, strong smell could be a sign of infection (*see pages 80-83*).

LUMPS AND BUMPS

With adulthood and changes in your shape, you will probably start to develop a new awareness of your body. Every now and again, check for signs of anything different or out of the ordinary. For example, breasts normally feel uneven, and before and during a period they can feel larger than usual and more lumpy and tender. You can get to know your breasts by checking them each month at the same time just after your

> *I hate it when people wear loads of perfume or aftershave – I always think they must be covering up some other smell. If you wash, you shouldn't need all that stuff.*
>
> Gurinder, 17 years

HAVING A PAP TEST

You lie down on a flat surface with your knees bent and your feet together. You then let your knees drop to the side. The doctor or nurse inserts a speculum into your vagina. This metal instrument holds the vaginal walls apart while the examination is being carried out. It won't hurt, though it can feel cold and you may feel pressure. A spatula is inserted through the speculum and scrapes cells from the cervix. You may not feel this. The sample of cells is put on a glass slide and sent to a lab to be analyzed. Your doctor or the clinic will tell you when to call for results. Keep a note in your diary so that you remember to have another checkup (usually every three years).

CHECKING THE TESTES

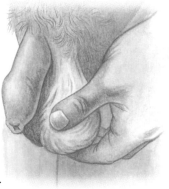

Testes should be examined regularly. The best time is just after a hot bath or shower, because the skin of the scrotum will be loose, making examination easy. Roll each testis between your thumb and fingers, gently moving the skin and feeling the entire surface. You are looking for changes in the texture, feel, size, and weight – the back of each testis is naturally lumpy (*see page 25*).

period. A painless lump or changes in skin texture are symptoms of one of the most common female cancers, though breast cancer is rare in young women. Early treatment improves the chances of successful treatment. If you note any changes or anything unusual, check with a doctor.

Cancer of the testes, while rare, is one of the most common cancers in young men. It can be cured if treated early. Regular checkups are a good idea. If you have a painless lump or swelling that wasn't there before, see a doctor to put your mind at ease.

THE PAP TEST

This is a screening procedure for cervical cancer that is carried out regularly on women who have ever been sexually active from the age of about 20, or within one to three years of having regular intercourse. This test is also known as a cervical smear. A doctor or nurse at a surgery or family planning clinic can do this. Abnormal cells on the cervix develop slowly and regular pap tests allow these to be treated, usually with lasers. Cervical cancer has been linked to early sexual activity, genital warts, and smoking.

❝ When my breasts first started, they were really lumpy, and I used to worry all the time that there was something wrong. ❞

Chrissie, 15 years

CHECKING THE BREASTS

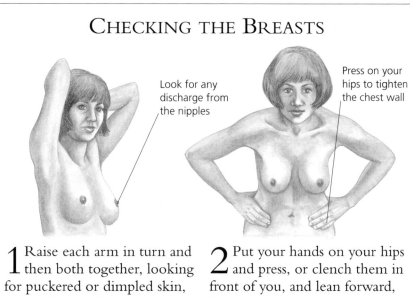

Look for any discharge from the nipples

Press on your hips to tighten the chest wall

1 Raise each arm in turn and then both together, looking for puckered or dimpled skin, or any changes in the nipples.

2 Put your hands on your hips and press, or clench them in front of you, and lean forward, looking for changes.

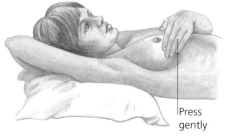

Press gently

3 Move your fingers over the entire surface of each breast. If you have large breasts, support them with the other hand. Feel for lumps and any changes in skin texture.

PERSONAL HYGIENE ESSENTIALS

For girls
■ Wipe from front to back after a bowel movement, to avoid spreading germs forward from the anus.
■ See your doctor if you have a different-smelling or colored discharge: you might have an infection that could be treated *(see pages 80-83).*
■ Don't use douches or vaginal deodorants: they are unnecessary and can irritate the vagina and cause infection.
■ Wash the vaginal area daily but avoid soaping between the vaginal lips, because soap may irritate the vulva.
■ Take regular baths or showers during your period.
For boys
■ If you are uncircumcised, pull your foreskin back to wash away the secretions (called smegma) that may accumulate underneath it.
■ Take regular baths or showers.
■ See your doctor if there is discharge from your penis.

Diseases and infections

Those who are sexually active can pass on or pick up a sexually transmitted disease (STD), so it is essential to take precautions. Sex is never free of the risk of unplanned pregnancy or an infection. Every sexually active person must be responsible and practice safer sex.

HOW DO YOU KNOW YOU'VE BEEN INFECTED?

Both sexes may have burning soreness or itching on or around the genitals, pain or discomfort when passing urine, or lumps, sores, blisters, or warts on or around the genitals. Men may have a clear or white discharge from the penis. Women's vaginal fluid may become heavier, change color, or have an unpleasant smell. Women may need to urinate more frequently. Sometimes, however, women have no symptoms.

Infections that are not sexually transmitted can cause similar symptoms, and sometimes infections don't cause symptoms at all. So if someone you've had sex with tells you that they have an infection, you should visit a doctor or a clinic, even if you have no symptoms.

VISITING A CLINIC

Clinics that treat sexually transmitted diseases may be independent or part of a hospital complex; call your local hospital or consult the telephone directory to find out where the nearest one is (*see pages 92-93*). Anything you tell the doctor or the clinic is confidential, but part of their job is to try to stop infections from spreading. They may ask you the names of your sexual partners, so that they can be contacted and treated. This can be done anonymously.

If you are worried about HIV (*see page 84*), the doctor or clinic can help you decide whether to have a test. If your family doctor does the test, it goes in your medical files. You might need to give someone access to these and not want them to know about the test. A test at a clinic is confidential.

WHAT HAPPENS AT A CLINIC?

At many independently run clinics, you don't need an appointment – you can walk in. The staff won't criticize you or give you a lecture. You will be examined and given tests, including a blood test. Once the disease or infection is identified – some results are given right away while others may take a few days – you will be given a course of treatment. Always finish any course of treatment, even if the symptoms

---

It was my first sexual experience and I was sure I'd gotten a sexually transmitted disease. It turned out to be just an irritation and the ointment cleared the itching up in 24 hours.

Pippa, 16 years

SAFER SEX

■ Always use a condom to protect your own and your partner's sexual health.
■ Remember that a condom only reduces the risk, it doesn't eliminate it.
■ Casual sex or a lot of partners increases the chances of meeting someone with a sexually transmitted disease.
■ If a partner or ex-partner tells you they think they have an STD, seek medical advice, even if you have no symptoms.
■ Alcohol and drugs can make you less careful than you should be about sex and more inclined to take chances.

go before your medication is gone, otherwise some germs may reinfect you. Many of those tested find out they have no disease.

WHY GO FOR TREATMENT?

With the exception of HIV *(see pages 84-85)*, STDs can be treated. Sometimes a disease or an infection does clear up by itself, but without treatment it can reappear. An untreated one can also spread, causing permanent damage to both you and your partner's health, and you may pass it on to someone else in the meantime. Some STDs can affect your chances of having children. Treatment is easiest if it is started early.

People who think they have caught a sexually transmitted disease often feel frightened or ashamed. They may feel too embarrassed to go to a clinic or see their doctor. Don't worry. Doctors and clinics deal with these problems all the time and will understand your feelings.

It can be difficult to tell someone that you have passed an infection on to them, or that you have an infection you could only have caught from them. But it is essential that your sexual partners know: they might have no symptoms and no idea that they have an STD. A clinic may be able to trace people for you and inform them anonymously.

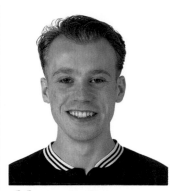

I thought I had something really awful and I was seriously sick, but the clinic gave me antibiotics, and it cleared up in couple of weeks.

Craig, 16 years

SYMPTOMS

If you notice anything different around your genitals and you are sexually active, then you may have a sexually transmitted disease. Refer to the following pages for a list of common infections and diseases that can affect the sexual organs. Common symptoms include:

- a white or different discharge from the penis – chlamydia, gonorrhea, NSU
- itching around the genitals – genital herpes, pubic lice, yeast infection
- sore, itchy genitals – vaginitis, yeast infection
- pain when urinating – chlamydia, gonorrhea, NSU
- lumps, sores, warts or blisters around the genitals – genital herpes, genital warts, syphilis
- an unusual discharge (frothy or yellow, for example) from the vagina – bacterial vaginosis, chlamydia, gonorrhea, yeast infection, trichomoniasis, vaginitis

- an unpleasant, smelly discharge – bacterial vaginosis, trichomoniasis
- frequent and/or painful urination – cystitis
- abdominal pain and tenderness – pelvic inflammatory disease

IF IN DOUBT

Practicing safer sex *(see left)* is a way to reduce the risk of a sexually transmitted disease, but if you suffer any of the symptoms listed above, it is best to abstain from any sexual contact until you have visited your doctor or a clinic to find out whether there is a problem or not. About half of the people who visit clinics have no sexually transmitted disease.

VAGINAL DISCHARGE

It is normal to have some vaginal discharge – this is the way the vagina cleans and lubricates itself *(see page 14)*. Normally, this discharge is colorless and doesn't smell, although it dries to leave a yellow or brownish stain on underwear. If it begins to have a bad smell, or to look different, perhaps frothy, this may indicate infection. Leaving a tampon in for too long can cause a foul-smelling vaginal discharge *(see Toxic shock, page 65)*.

DISEASES AND INFECTIONS

NAME	SYMPTOMS	TREATMENT
Bacterial vaginosis	A grayish, frothy discharge with a fishy odor, caused by a bacteria naturally present in womens' bodies that has multiplied out of control. Men can also have the germs, but usually without symptoms.	Antibiotic drugs or creams to insert into the vagina. If untreated, this infection may cause fertility problems.
Chlamydia	In men, pain on passing urine and a discharge from the penis. Women may have a vaginal discharge or no symptoms. There may be pelvic pain during sex.	Antibiotics. If untreated, this could lead to infertility and other problems in women and men.
Cystitis	Frequent and painful urination, maybe only a trickle, which may smell strong and contain traces of blood. This is an infection of the bladder caused by bacteria that are naturally present in the body. Cystitis is common in women, because a woman's urethra is short and the bacteria are able to reach the bladder from the rectum (see page 15). If a woman has strenuous sexual intercourse, this can trigger a state called "mechanical stress," resulting in cystitis. Men have a longer urethra, so cystitis in men is rare.	Drinking plenty of water (with a teaspoon of bicarbonate of soda added to each glass) at the first sign of the symptoms can help keep your urine flowing. Drink about two glasses of liquids every hour. If symptoms do not disappear, or you are uncomfortable, your doctor may prescribe antibiotics.
Genital herpes	Tenderness, tingling, and itching of the genitals, followed by blisters, which may burst to form painful sores. There is often pain on urinating, and sometimes a feeling of illness and a raised temperature. This disease is caused by the herpes simplex II virus. It can be caught through intercourse and is different from the herpes simplex I virus that causes cold sores on the mouth. The first outbreak usually clears up in about two weeks, but the virus stays in the body and may lead to further outbreaks.	The virus cannot be killed, but antiviral drugs and painkillers help heal sores and reduce pain during attacks. Sex must be avoided, or condoms used, during attacks. Women who have genital herpes should have regular Pap smears because there may be an increased risk of cervical cancer.
Genital warts	Soft warts appear on and around the anus, the penis, or the entrance to the vagina and cervix. They may go undetected because they are small, or disappear of their own accord. These are also called venereal warts. Untreated, they may multiply rapidly, so early treatment is advisable.	They are removed by repeated application of a lotion or by surgery, but they tend to recur. Any woman who has had them, or whose partner has had them, should be sure to have an annual Pap smear (see page 78,), because of the link between genital warts and an increased risk of cervical cancer.
Gonorrhea	Men suffer pain on passing urine and have a discharge from the penis. Women contract the disease more rarely, and may have a vaginal discharge, or no symptoms.	Antibiotics. If untreated, the disease can cause infertility in men and women, so a woman's partner must be checked, too.
HIV and AIDs (see pages 84-86)		

NAME	SYMPTOMS	TREATMENT
Nonspecific urethritis (NSU)	This inflammation of the urethra mostly affects men, who may have pain on passing urine or a discharge from the penis: these symptoms can be mild. Women may have a slight vaginal discharge or, often, no symptoms. This is one of the most common sexually transmitted diseases, called nonspecific because its cause cannot always be identified.	Antibiotics. If untreated, infections can cause serious complications such as a rare form of arthritis. In women, there may be later complications such as pelvic inflammatory disease.
Pelvic inflammatory disease (PID)	Symptoms include abdominal pain and tenderness, often immediately after or during sex. Periods may become irregular and painful. There may also be fever, backache, and vomiting. This is an infection of the female reproductive system. It cannot be passed on to sexual partners, but it is often a result of an untreated infection such as chlamydia or gonorrhea.	Antibiotics and, in some cases, painkillers and bed rest. If the woman has an IUD in place, it should be removed if the infection does not respond to treatment. If left untreated, chronic pelvic pain or an abcess can develop.
Pubic lice (crabs)	Bloodsucking, crablike parasites, the size of a pinhead, which live in the pubic hair, where they cause itching. Pubic lice are sometimes passed on by sharing bedding, clothes, and towels, although usually by sexual contact.	The white, shiny eggs cannot be removed by normal washing: a special over-the-counter medication or antibiotic may be prescribed. Towels, clothes, and bedding must be washed in very hot water to prevent reinfection.
Syphilis	The first sign of syphilis is a painless, but very infectious, sore at the site of infection, commonly the genitalia, rectum, tongue, or lips. This heals on its own in a few weeks, but the germs remain in the body and develop.	Antibiotics. If untreated, the disease will progress to cause a rash, mouth sores, and general aching. If not treated, the disease can be fatal.
Trichomoniasis	A frothy, yellowish, foul-smelling vaginal discharge in women. Men may suffer symptoms similar to those for NSU, but often have no symptoms. Trich, as it is known, is caused by parasites that infect the vagina in women, and the urethra in men.	Antibiotics.
Vaginitis	Irritation and sometimes discharge. It can be caused by various bacteria, usually thrush, trichomoniasis, or bacterial vaginosis. Allergies to spermicides or to scented soaps can also cause inflammation.	Antifungal or antibiotic drugs, depending on the cause, or avoiding the cause of the irritation.
Yeast infection	A white, curdy discharge, genital itching, redness and swelling of the vulva, and soreness on passing urine. This is not caused by sexual contact, but by a yeast or fungus that is naturally present in the vagina. This infection is very common in women. A woman can pass it to a sexual partner through sexual contact, although this is rare. The glans of the penis may become inflamed.	Antibiotics and creams. A yeast infection thrives in warm and airless conditions, so if a woman has an attack, it is wise to wear cotton underwear and avoid pantyhose and tight pants.

HIV and AIDS

HIV is a virus that causes the illness known as AIDS. Anyone can contract this virus through unprotected sexual intercourse with an infected person or by using infected needles. It is estimated that around 12 million people worldwide have contracted HIV.

The immune system

The body has an immune system that is its defense against infection. However, if the human immunodeficiency virus (HIV) enters the body, the cells in the body's immune system are invaded and cannot destroy the virus. HIV stays alive within the cells of the immune system, and may lie dormant there for years. At present, there is no known way to kill this virus once it enters the body. A blood test will detect HIV. If there is HIV, the person is said to be HIV positive. Being HIV positive does not make people ill. Someone with HIV may look and feel well, and stay this way for a long time – often for years. But they are infectious to others, and will be for the rest of their lives.

The onset of AIDS

When HIV is active, the infected cells in the immune system die, and the virus is released into the blood to infect other cells. As the immune system is weakened, the person loses weight, tires easily, and becomes more vulnerable to all sorts of infections, such as skin disorders, ulcers, yeast infection, and diarrhea. Eventually, serious problems, such as herpes, tuberculosis, pneumonia, and cancer, develop.

When a person becomes ill in this way, they are said to be suffering from acquired immune deficiency syndrome, or AIDS. Once a person reaches this final stage of the disease, they usually die of a major infection within a year or two.

How does HIV spread?

HIV is found only in bodily fluids, and of these blood, semen, saliva, and vaginal fluids have been shown to transmit infection. The virus enters the body through a sore or cut in the skin, or an injection, or through the membranes that line the mouth, the vagina, or the anus. A baby can contract HIV from its mother through the placenta in the uterus, or possibly through breast milk after birth.

The virus cannot survive for long outside the human body. It is perfectly safe to live with someone who has HIV or

---

❝ When my dad told me my uncle was HIV positive, I just couldn't believe it. I didn't know what to say to him at first, but he acted just the same, so I do, too. ❞

Ben, 12 years

HOW HIV IS SPREAD

It can be spread by bodily fluids through:
- Unprotected sex.
- An open wound.
- Shared needles.
- Mother to unborn child.

It cannot be spread by:
- Toilet seats, showers.
- Food, dishes, etc.
- Coughs, sneezes, sweat, tears.
- Hugs, handshakes.
- Insect bites.

AIDS, to share their food, to use the same silverware and dishes, to touch or hug them, and even to sleep in the same bed as them. It is not safe to exchange bodily fluids through unprotected sex, or by sharing toothbrushes, razors, or, in the case of drug users, hypodermic syringes, with anyone who is, or may be, HIV positive. Doing so puts one at serious risk of contracting HIV.

THE SEARCH FOR A SOLUTION

There is no real cure for even the mildest virus, such as the common cold. At present, there is no cure for AIDS and no vaccine against it. Various drugs have been tried in the hope that they can slow down the progress of AIDS; however, the search still goes on for a cure.

The other area of research is the attempt to find a vaccine. Worldwide vaccination for smallpox wiped out the disease in this century: if a vaccine against HIV can be developed, AIDS might also be overcome.

SAFER SEX

Everyone can avoid doing things that put them at risk. Many people have already changed their behavior to reduce the risks of infection; many still take risks, however. While you can never completely eliminate the chances of catching any infection, you can do a lot to protect yourself against being infected by HIV.

Kissing, touching, hugging, or mutual masturbation are usually safe, unless open sores are present. Oral sex is slightly more risky, because bleeding gums and mouth sores are quite common and can provide a point of entry for the virus (*see page 51*).

Sexual intercourse is still the most common means of infection. There is a higher risk with anal intercourse, because the lining of the anus tears more easily than that of the vagina, providing a way in for the virus. The risk can be reduced during intercourse by wearing a condom (*see pages 60-62*).

MINIMIZING THE RISKS

Most people know that unprotected sex carries risks and that the more sexual partners you have, the higher the chances that one of them is HIV positive. But even with people you know, there is a risk. Whatever risks your partner takes or has taken in the past, you are taking too. Anything that involves blood can be risky: drug addicts who inject drugs have contracted HIV. Addicts who share needles or use dirty needles are putting themselves at risk.

Everyone should avoid sharing items such as razors, and

> *He made such a fuss when I asked him to put on a condom – you'd think I was asking him to come to bed wearing his boots. He put it on, though.*
>
> Debbie, 17 years

LIVING WITH HIV

Many people with HIV stay well for years. The people around them may never know that they are HIV positive. People who are ignorant about AIDS are often frightened and can be cruel, so people who are HIV positive may be happier if only those close to them know. If you know someone with HIV, you can still be their friend. Just treat them normally, not fussing over them too much, but remember that they may sometimes tire easily or get depressed. If they want to talk about it, encourage them, and listen sympathetically. If they don't want to talk about it, accept that, too.

even toothbrushes – people often have mouth sores or minor cuts on their gums without even being aware of them. Tattooing and ear-piercing could also carry a small risk if instruments are not sterilized: ask about the hygiene methods used (*see below*). Having a blood transfusion should no longer be dangerous, because blood is now carefully screened.

When the disease first appeared in the developed world, most of its victims were gay or bisexual men, so some people used to think that AIDS was a disease solely of gay men. This is not true. This prejudice can encourage heterosexuals to think that they are safe. It is better to behave in ways that will reduce the risks for everyone instead of assuming that if you are female or heterosexual, you are unlikely to be infected.

HAVING AN HIV TEST

If you are worried about HIV and AIDS, you should talk to a special counselor in a clinic or contact a special hotline (*see pages 92-93*). Many clinics will not test you without this counseling, because the implications of the test are greater than people imagine.

The test is *not* for AIDS. The test determines whether you have antibodies to HIV in your blood. Usually, the antibodies appear within six weeks of infection, but they can take up to six months to show up, so you may test negative but be asked to return for another test in six months. During this time, you should not do anything that puts you or any partner at risk.

QUESTIONS AND ANSWERS

Someone told me I shouldn't have my ears pierced because I might get HIV from the needle they use. Can this really happen?
Nicky, 14 years

This could happen if an unsterilized needle was used, which might have been previously used on someone who had HIV or AIDS. The same is true for the needles used for tattoos and acupuncture. But if you go to a reputable jeweler or store, there should be no risk: their needles should be sterile, or they should be using disposable needles. Don't be embarrassed to ask about hygiene methods before you have the piercing done, and if you're not happy, go elsewhere.

What does an HIV test involve, and if there's no cure, what's the point in anyone taking it?
Pete, 16 years

A small blood sample is taken and tested. The results are available in a few days – in some clinics on the same day. If the result is positive, the person infected will need to take steps to avoid passing the virus on to anyone else. They should tell anyone who needs to know: their partner, their doctor, their dentist, and their family. Because it can take from six to eight weeks from the time of infection for the antibodies to appear, the test is usually not considered reliable until six months after exposure to the infection.

PROBLEM AREAS

- Sex and the law
- Child sexual abuse
- Sexual harassment
- Rape

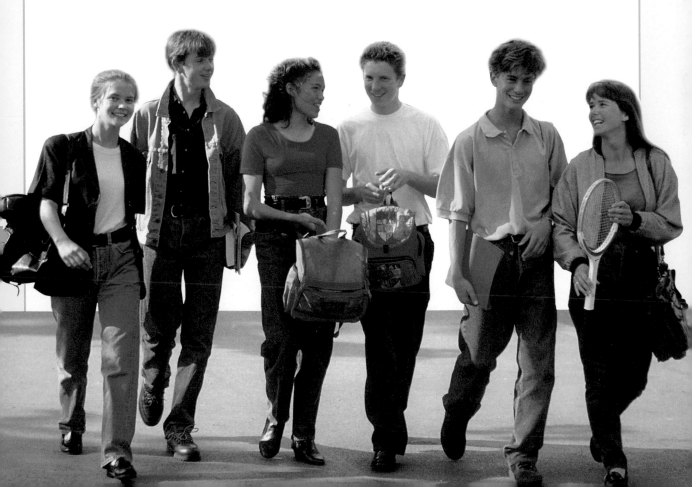

Sex and the law

Whatever happens to your body should only happen with your consent, and because you want it to happen. There are laws designed to protect people from abuse by others.

THE AGE OF CONSENT

The law protects children until they are old enough to make their own decisions about sex. The age at which you are considered old enough to do this is called the age of consent. If you are under the age of consent *(see page 44)* and someone has sex with you, even if you agree to it, they are committing an offense. The age of consent varies from state to state.

SEXUAL OFFENSES

Some behavior is always against the law. Incest (sex with close relations such as a parent or an uncle or aunt) is always illegal, regardless of age. Anything that offends or harms others, such as sexual harassment *(see opposite),* or that forces someone to have intercourse or commit a sexual act against their will *(see page 91),* is also against the law.

PORNOGRAPHY

Pornography is any material designed to arouse the viewer sexually. Some people claim that lightly clad people in advertisements are pornographic, while others claim that they are harmless. In most countries, the law allows some kinds of material, but bans others. "Hard-core" porn shows sexual acts with violence and depicts its subjects as objects to be dominated or humiliated. In most countries, such material is illegal.

Pornography has been shown to affect people's attitudes; it can change the way that we view other people. People in real life are unlikely to be as willing or as adventurous.

PROSTITUTION

Prostitution is the sale of sex, by men or women. In most countries, it is either illegal, or made very difficult by laws that a prostitute cannot avoid breaking. Few of these laws protect the prostitute, who leads a dangerous life, exposed to the risks of HIV infection and other sexually transmitted infections, and of violence. In the US and Canada, prostitution is illegal.

Child sexual abuse

Child sexual abuse is any activity in which children are used by other people for sexual pleasure. It includes not only intercourse, but any kind of sexual touching.

WHO ABUSES?

Usually the abuser is a friend of the family, a relation, or someone known to the child. Sometimes a child is abused by a parent, a sibling, a stepparent, or stepbrothers or stepsisters.

It is difficult to know exactly how many children are, or have been, abused. When adults are questioned about their childhood, a large number (and twice as many women as men) say that they were abused. Thousands of children call telephone hotlines every year to confide that they have been, or are being, sexually abused.

WHAT IS ABUSE?

If you're not certain about what someone is doing, or whether it is abuse or not, ask yourself the following questions to help you make up your mind. Does what is happening make you feel uncomfortable? Are you being sworn to secrecy so that nobody else knows about it? Are they doing it for their pleasure, with no regard for how you feel? Do they threaten you or ignore you if you try to stop them? Do they say that something bad will happen if you tell? If the answer to any of these questions is yes, then you are being abused.

WHAT SHOULD YOU DO?

No matter who is abusing you, try to tell an adult what is happening. Even though you feel fearful about what will happen, telling someone is the best thing to do. This is easy advice to give, but it is often difficult to follow, especially if a member of your family is involved.

It is important for you to realize that when an adult abuses a child, it is *always* the adult's fault, *never* the child's. It may take time for you to summon up the courage to tell someone what is happening, but nothing is likely to change unless you do.

A parent is the best person to tell, if you can. If you can't, tell a grandparent or another close relative whom you trust, a mature friend, or a sympathetic teacher at school. Or you can call one of the telephone hotlines or organizations *(see pages 92-93)* and talk in confidence to a specially trained counselor. They can advise you on the next step to take.

WHAT HAPPENS NEXT?

If the police or social services are told that a child is being sexually abused at home, the first thing they must do is make sure that the child is safe. If necessary, the authorities remove the child from the home, at least for a time. This "breathing space" gives everyone a chance to decide what should be done for the best interest of the child and to seek professional help for both the child and the abuser, if possible.

The police will decide whether to charge the person concerned or not. They must check on everyone's story and collect evidence. Sometimes they can't bring charges – this doesn't mean that a crime has not been committed. If the case does go to court, the victim may have to appear in court and give evidence. By telling someone, the abused person may have prevented the abuser from doing the same thing again.

Reporting sexual abuse is a difficult thing to do, but it is necessary. It can also be traumatic, and for this reason, most victims find counseling helpful.

Sexual harassment

This is unwanted pestering of a sexual nature. It doesn't have to be physical – comments, whistling, or obscene telephone calls are also sexual harassment.

WHAT TO DO ABOUT IT

Sexual harassment is not about attraction, it is about belittling someone. It is often done by people in positions of power. If you have been harassed, remember that it was not your fault. You are not alone: many people are harassed every day. Even if you are scared, don't keep it to yourself, but tell someone you trust. Sharing the experience will often make you feel better. Most harassment is illegal, so report incidents to someone in authority or to the police so that the perpetrator can be caught.

If the sexual harassment happens at school, take the names of any witnesses and tell a parent and a teacher or the principal. If your complaint is ignored, inform the board of education; if the harassment involves a criminal offense, notify the police. If you feel you have a valid complaint, do not be persuaded to drop the matter. You may have to sign a statement naming your harasser in order to have any action taken.

WHISTLES AND COMMENTS

Harassment of this sort is common. You may feel angered and humiliated, but depending on where you are and who you are with, you can either try to ignore it – responding may encourage the harasser – or be assertive and tell the harasser that you don't accept this behavior. If anything like this happens at school, report it. Students, and even teachers, sometimes comment on teenagers' physical development. If you don't like this, tell the person, and if they go on, report it. If someone makes unwanted sexual suggestions, tell them to stop, ask others if it has happened to them, and report it to someone in authority.

FLASHERS AND PEEPING TOMS

Flashers are men who expose their penises in public. Get away as fast as you can. In all cases, tell a parent or teacher and the police. Flashing is a crime.

Voyeurs are people who try to watch others when they are undressing or naked, or having sex. They are also known as "peeping toms." If you ever see someone spying on you, tell a parent, and report it to the police. Voyeurism is a crime.

UNWANTED TOUCHING

Crowded places, such as trains or buses, give some people the chance to touch or rub themselves against you. Draw attention to what is going on by loudly telling the offender to stop, and tell a parent or other adult as soon as you can. Contact the police: this kind of harassment is a crime.

OBSCENE TELEPHONE CALLS

Also called nuisance, or dirty, phone calls, these are upsetting and illegal. Callers may be silent, or ask intimate questions, or make sexual threats. If you receive an obscene call, put the phone down calmly – don't slam it down. Don't talk to the caller, and never give your name. Tell a parent, and contact the police and the telephone company. Calls can usually be traced easily, so if the caller persists, they can be caught and prosecuted.

CURB CRAWLERS

Curb crawlers are drivers who harass pedestrians by driving slowly behind them, sometimes making obscene suggestions. Ignore any comments and walk away from the car. If possible, memorize the license plate and make of car and pass the information on to the police. Curb crawling is an offense.

Rape

If someone forces you to have sex against your will, it is rape – whether you are a man or a woman. Other forms of sexual attack are known as indecent assault.

WHAT IS RAPE?

Rape is a frightening and horrible experience, and often rape victims feel guilty, even though they have done nothing wrong. They may feel dirty, as though they have been somehow "spoiled." Because of these feelings, the first reaction may be to tell nobody and to pretend that nothing has happened.

YOU MAY KNOW YOUR ATTACKER

Most rape victims know the person who rapes them. When a girl is raped by someone she knows, it is often called "date rape." Many such rapes happen at or after parties, when one (or both) of the people involved has had too much to drink. If the girl says no, and the boy insists, this is still rape. If she finally gives in, she may feel raped because she didn't want to do it, although the boy could claim that she had consented. There is sometimes a fine line, however, between date rape and sexual misunderstanding. Boys and girls often expect different things: each assumes that the other knows what they want (or don't want), but they can't read each other's signals. Girls must be clear about what they want and make it clear that they mean it when they say no. And boys have to accept and believe a no as readily as they would a yes.

WHAT TO DO IF YOU ARE RAPED

It isn't always easy to tell anyone, let alone the police. You may be afraid of the person who raped you, or fear you won't be believed. But, if you keep silent, it may be harder for you to get over what has happened. It also allows your attacker to go unpunished, and they may rape someone else. Tell your parents, a relative, or a close friend. They should report the rape to the police at once. You may be able to talk to a specially trained policewoman, who will make it as easy for you to talk as she can.

Even if you feel that you just want to forget the whole thing, it is sensible to collect some evidence. Forensic evidence, such as tiny fragments of skin under your nails, can be vital in securing a conviction. It is important that you be examined, either by a police doctor or by your own doctor, within 24 hours of the rape. The doctor's report is essential evidence if the police are to prosecute your attacker.

It will help you if you can talk about it to someone else, especially someone who has had a similar experience. Contact a rape crisis center or a telephone hotline about this *(see pages 92 93),* or ask your doctor to refer you to a counselor.

Useful addresses

ABUSE & ASSAULT

Childhelp USA, Inc.
6463 Independence Avenue
Woodland Hills, CA 91367
Tel: 1-800-4-A-CHILD

Local Rape Crisis Centers (consult telephone directory)

National Committee for Prevention of Child Abuse
332 S. Michigan Ave, Ste. 1600
Chicago, IL 60604-4357
Tel: (312) 663-3520

National Council on Child Abuse and Family Violence
1155 Connecticut Avenue NW
Ste. 400
Washington, DC 20036
Tel: 1-800-222-2000

ADOPTION

Adoption Families of America
3333 Highway 100 North
Minneapolis, MN 55422
Tel: (612) 535-4829

National Adoption Center
1500 Walnut Street
Ste. 1701
Philadelphia, PA 19102
Tel: 1-800-TO-ADOPT

National Committee for Adoption
1930 17th St. NW
Washington, DC 20009-6207
Tel: (202) 328-8072 (National Adoption Hotline)

COUNSELING

American Psychiatric Association
1400 K Street NW
Washington, DC 20005
Tel: (202) 682-6000

Anxiety Disorders Association of America
6000 Executive Boulevard, Ste. 513
Rockville, MD 20852
Tel: (301) 231-9350

The Coalition on Sexuality and Disability
122 East 23rd Street
New York, NY 10010
Tel: (212) 242-3900

National Depressive and Manic Depressive Association
730 North Franklin, Ste. 501
Chicago, IL 60610
Tel: (312) 642-0049

National Mental Health Association
1021 Prince Street
Alexandria, VA 22314-2971
Tel: 1-800-969-NMHA

DRUGS

Alcoholics Anonymous
General Service
475 Riverside Drive
New York, NY 10115
Tel: (212) 870-3400

American Cancer Society
1599 Clifton Road NE
Atlanta, GA 30329
Tel: (404) 320-3333

Families Anonymous
PO Box 528
Van Nuys, CA 91408
Tel: 1-800-736-9805

National Council on Alcoholism and Drug Dependence
12 West 21st Street
New York, NY 10010
Tel: 1-800-NCA-CALL

800-Cocaine
PO Box 100
Summit, NJ 07902-0100
Tel: 1-800-262-2463

EATING DISORDERS

The American Anorexia/Bulimia Association
c/o Regent Hospital
425 E. 61st Street
6th fl.
New York, NY 10021
Tel: (212) 891-8686

ANAD-National Association of Anorexia Nervosa and Associated Disorders
PO Box 7
Highland Park, IL 60035
Tel: (708) 831-3438

FAMILY RELATIONS

Family Resource Coalition
200 South Michigan Avenue
Ste. 1520
Chicago, IL 60604
Tel: (312) 341-0900

Family Service America, Inc.
11700 West Lake Park Drive
Milwaukee, WI 53224
Tel: (414) 359-1040

National Council on Family Relations
3989 Central Avenue NE, Ste. 550
Minneapolis, MN 55421
Tel: (612) 781-9331

Parents without Partners, Inc.
c/o Smith Bucklin Associates
401 North Michigan Avenue
Chicago, ILL 60611
Tel: (312) 644-6610

MEDICAL CONCERNS

National Alliance of Breast Cancer Organizations
1180 Avenue of the Americas
New York, NY 10036
Tel: (212) 719-0154

National Herpes Hotline
Tel: (919) 361-8488

National STD Hotline
Tel: 1-800-227-8922

SIECUS (Sex Information and Education Council of the US)
130 West 42nd Street
Ste. 2500
New York, NY 10036
Tel: (212) 819-9770

Local Hospital Clinics

AIDS Hotlines

PREGNANCY & CONTRACEPTION

American College of Obstetricians and Gynecologists (ACOG)
409 12th Street SW
Washington, DC 20024-2188
Contact : Adolescence
Tel: (202) 638-5577

Informed Homebirth
PO Box 3675
Ann Arbor, MI 48106
Tel: (313) 662-6857

National Abortion Federation
1436 U Street NW, Ste. 103
Washington, DC 20009
Tel: 1-800-772-9100

National Organization of Adolescent Pregnancy and Parenting
4421A East-West Highway
Bethesda, MD 20814
Tel: (301) 913-0378

Planned Parenthood Federation of America
810 Seventh Avenue
New York, NY 10019
Tel: 1-800-829-PPFA

GENERAL

U.S. Department of Health and Human Services
Public Health Service
Centers for Disease Control and Prevention
National Center for Health Statistics
6525 Belcrest Road
Hyattsville, MD 20782

Index

Acknowledgments

Dorling Kindersley and the authors would like to thank:
Sashola Mahoney, Mark Noble and Candida Ross-MacDonald
for help with the text; the young men and women for being
models; Antony Heller and Maryann Rogers for production
assistance; Camela Decaire for editorial assistance.

Special photography
Antonia Deutsch

Illustration
Coral Mula

Index
Jane Parker

Picture research
Clive Webster

Additional photography
Stephen Bartholomew, Andy Crawford, Tim Ridley,
Hanya Chlala (jacket front)

Picture credits
Comstock: 44, 46; /R. Michael Stuckey 3b
The Image Bank: /Werner Bokelberg 9
Oxford Scientific Films, Mantis Wildlife Films: 70c, 71tl
Pictor International: 30, 40
Science Photo Library: 66, 67; /Andy Walker, Midland Fertility
Services: 71ct, 71b; /CNRI: 71tr; /John Walsh 70b
Telegraph Colour Library: 87; /R. Chapple 32, 37b; /Marco
Polo 33b; /Paul von Stroheim 87
Zefa: 3r, 29, 34, 45, 77; /Norman 2; /Wartenberg 3

tlt=top b=bottom l=left r=right